Ramata Yakaré TRAORE

Knowledge, Attitudes and Prevention Practices of Populations

Ramata Yakaré TRAORE

Knowledge, Attitudes and Prevention Practices of Populations

Baco-Djicoroni Health Area

ScienciaScripts

Cover image: www.ingimage.com

This book is a translation from the original published under ISBN 978-620-6-70691-5.

Publisher:
Sciencia Scripts
is a trademark of
Dodo Books Indian Ocean Ltd. and OmniScriptum S.R.L publishing group

120 High Road, East Finchley, London, N2 9ED, United Kingdom
Str. Armeneasca 28/1, office 1, Chisinau MD-2012, Republic of Moldova, Europe
Printed at: see last page
ISBN: 978-620-7-95169-7

Contents

Tribute to Dr Mamadou B Coulibaly

Dear Master,

You left before us, far too soon, and you remind us that our lives here are nothing. I am very happy to have shared a part of your life with you. You had the art of cultivating excellence, and you inspired us to love research even more. You were a real pillar for your family and your colleagues. Your departure leaves a void in the hearts of all those who worked with you. On a day-to-day basis, you were the man for the job. I know that this text will not be able to express everything I want to say to you, but I would like everyone who has the chance to read this book to know that you were a great man and a great researcher who served the world and Mali in particular.

Rest in peace Le Génie

DEDICATIONS AND THANKS

DEDICACES

To Almighty and Merciful Allah!

For guiding me and giving me the necessary strength and courage to carry out this modest work.

Thank you for the grace you have bestowed on me, grant me your blessing so that I may be wise, so that my days may be multiplied and the years of my life increased in peace, the better to praise you.

To the prophet Mohamed (peace be upon him).

May God's peace and blessings be upon you and your companions. Our respect and gratitude for all you have done for humanity.

I dedicate this work :

To my father Tiémoko Dialla TRAORE

More than a father, you're a role model for me; you're the one who has always gone out of his way to put his children in the best possible conditions. I can never thank you enough. You gave me everything in life; everything I am today I owe to you. You always wanted me to become a doctor like your sister, my namesake (may she rest in peace), and well, I'm almost there DAD.

Thank you for your support, advice, encouragement and everything you do for my sons. This work is yours because of your immense qualities as a father. May Almighty God grant you a long and healthy life. I love you with all my heart.

To my mother Coumba COULIBALY

The sweetest and most wonderful of all mothers. You've always believed in me, Mum, and fought so hard to make me what I am today. I am eternally indebted to you for the most important thing of all: life. You've been through so much in the past but you've always been able to pick yourself up and move on. Today your patience and efforts have paid off; you're in the best possible condition, thanks to the grace of God. I see the fighting spirit in you and I'll do everything I can to be like you.

Thank you for all your advice, which has enabled me to be dignified in everything I do and always keep my head up in any situation. Thank you for making my sons yours. This work is also yours; may God grant you a long and healthy life! Amen to that!

To my husband Dr Mody KOUMA

You have given me so much support in my studies; it's also thanks to you that I've reached this stage. The love, patience and calm that you have always shown me have encouraged me to go ahead with this work. May God allow us to realise all our dreams and may our union be preserved. Thank you for everything.

To my brother Abdoulaye Fadiala TRAORE

As the only son, you always took care of the whole family. I pray to God that he will keep you on good terms with your colleagues in France and that he will keep you with us for a long time.

Thank you for being there despite the distance.

To my sisters Fatoumata Fily TRAORE; Aminata Sokona TRAORE and Oumou Tiémoko TRAORE

You have always supported me in my choices and encouraged me to make them, and I can't tell you how much respect and love I have for you. You have given me everything in life, thank you. This work is the fruit of our fraternity. May the good Lord continue to work in your lives.

To my sons Bréhima KOUMA and Tiémoko KOUMA

It's to see you succeed that I fight every day of my life; you are my joy in life. Your arrival in this world has been an opportunity for me to show everyone that having a child is no obstacle to academic success. Having you as a son fills my heart with pride; long live my babies; continue to be assiduous at school; stick to the education I give you and always follow the right path. I love you all.

TO THE LATE BAKARY CAMARA

After the baccalauréat, only 2 of us wanted to go to medical school with the aim of one day becoming a doctor, but we failed to pass the numerus clausus together, so fate wanted us to continue our journey together until your last day. You weren't just my classmate, you were my best friend. In year 6e , I lost you forever as a result of a road accident; the pain is still with me, but I live with it and pray to the good Lord that he will welcome you into his vast paradise and that your soul may rest in eternal peace. To God my best friend Bassaro!

Acknowledgements

To my uncles: Makan TRAORE and Sadio Mady TRAORE

My second dads, thank you for all your advice, encouragement and your love for me. This thesis is also yours.

To my aunts : Fanta MINTA, Rokia SOW, Fatim KEITA

I would like to express my deepest gratitude to all of you, dear aunts, for your generous blessings to each of us in this work.

To my cousins: Makan TRAORE, Mariam Fily TRAORE, Hawa Nahan TRAORE, Mariam TRAORE, Mohamed Fadiala TRAORE, Fatim KEITA, Lountandy KEITA, Haby MARIKO, Adiara Yakaré TRAORE, Ousmane TRAORE.

Thank you to all of you for your encouragement and for the great times we've had together.

To my childhood friends: Oumou DIARRA, Nana SAMAKE, Rokia DIARRA, Mariam BALLO.

True friends always recognise each other in difficult times. In many circumstances you have proved to me that beyond friendship you are sisters. Without you, I would never have been able to carry out this work. It is yours. Rest assured of my eternal loyalty. May this fraternity remain between us so that our dearest wishes come true. Amen to that!

To my in-laws

This thesis is sincerely dedicated to all of you, old and young, who are or have been part of this family. Please find here my most sincere thanks.

To the TRAORE family: Dr Sanachi TRAORE and Dr Nansa KANTE

You have been invaluable in helping me to complete this work. May God grant you a long and healthy life. Thank you very much.

To my presentation group: Dr Adama DOUMBIA, Dr Boubacar DIALLO, Dr Ousmane DIANE, Dr Cheickna Hamala TEMBELY, Dr Daouda GOITA, Aminata FOFANA.

You taught me to study harder; the competition between us in the group and our desire to always surpass ourselves enabled us to persevere in our work, to do better and to be among the best in our class. Please accept my sincere gratitude.

To my friends: Dr Lalla Mariam CISSE, Dr Fatoumata KASSE, Dr Nansa KANTE, Dr Moussa KONATE, Baba Elhaj CISSE, Dr Kourédja DIAKITE.

You've made my life at university so much easier. Thank you for all the moments of sharing.

May God protect you.

To my classmate: Aminata FOFANA

My unconditional classmate who has become my confidante and best friend over the years, you have always carried me in your heart and have always been there through good times and bad. I'll never be able to thank you enough for everything you've done for me. May the Almighty repay you a hundredfold and give you a long life.

To all the staff of the Baco-Djicoroni Cscom

Thank you for everything.

To the people of Baco-Djicoroni

Thank you for your contribution to the success of this project.

To all Target Malaria staff

From the director to the security guards, especially Dr Sidy Doumbia, thank you for the warm welcome and the respect you have shown me.

To all the staff of the Public Health Department

Thank you for your support in carrying out this work. I would also like to sincerely thank Bakara DICKO for everything.

To all FMOS teaching staff

I am delighted to have this opportunity to express my gratitude to you. Your dedicated teaching will remain a precious memory that will guide my professional life.

Yours sincerely

More than a medical school, for us it's a school for life.

To my beautiful country: MALI

In these difficult times that you are going through, you nonetheless make me experience this emotion and this joy that enlarges my heart. I hope that these crises will never shake your foundations.

God bless you!

At the 11[e] numerus clausus class

Thank you for all the wonderful years we've spent together.

To all those I have omitted to mention

I'm really sorry, but no human work can be perfect. I hold each and every one of you in my heart.

Chapter 1

INTRODUCTION

1. Introduction

Malaria is caused by parasites of the genus *Plasmodium* transmitted by female mosquitoes belonging to the genus Anopheles [1]. There are many species of *Plasmodium* (over 140), affecting various animal species, five of which are usually found in human pathology: *P. falciparum, P. vivax, P. malariae, P. ovale* and *P. knowlesi* [2]. Of these, *P. falciparum* and *P. vivax* have the highest prevalence, while *P. falciparum* is the most dangerous. *P. knowlesi* is a zoonotic species that can also infect humans [1].

In 1992, the World Health Organisation (WHO) declared in Amsterdam that malaria is a major threat to health and an obstacle to the socio-economic development of individuals, communities and nations [3].

Prevention is a major component of the fight against malaria. It focuses on vector control, chemoprevention and intermittent preventive treatment. Vector control is the principal means of preventing and reducing malaria transmission. If there is sufficient coverage of vector control interventions in a given area, the whole community would be protected. The WHO recommends effective vector control to protect populations at risk of contracting malaria. Two large-scale vector control strategies recommended by the WHO are effective in many situations: insecticide-treated mosquito nets (ITNs) and indoor residual spraying (IRS). IRS and ITNs have been shown to be effective in reducing malaria morbidity and mortality to some extent [4].

Vector control in Mali is guided by the national vector control strategy steered by the National Malaria Control Programme (PNLP). This strategy is based on universal coverage with long-lasting insecticide-treated nets (LLINs), capacity building, implementation of indoor residual spraying (IRS) in targeted districts, management of insecticide resistance and collaboration with the private sector. The 2018-2022 strategic plan aims to protect 80% of the population targeted by IRS, treat 95% of mosquito breeding sites and encourage regular use of LLINs by 80% of the population at risk by 2022 [5].

Insecticide-treated mosquito nets (ITNs) help to reduce contact between humans and vectors, thanks both to the physical barrier they create and to their insecticidal effect. General access and widespread use in the community mean that large numbers of mosquitoes can be killed, providing better protection for the population [6].

Indoor residual spraying is another highly effective way of rapidly reducing malaria transmission. Indoor residual spraying is used, usually once or twice a year. But to achieve significant community protection, a high level of coverage is required [6].

Malaria can also be prevented with anti-malarial drugs. Travellers can protect themselves with chemoprophylaxis that suppresses the blood stage of the malaria infection, preventing the disease from breaking out. Since 2012, the WHO has recommended seasonal malaria chemoprevention as a complementary malaria prevention strategy for the Sahel sub-region of Africa [7].

Chapter 2

ISSUES

2 Issues

In 2021, there will be an estimated 247 million cases of malaria worldwide, most of them (228 million or 95%) in Africa. The number of deaths due to malaria is estimated at 619,000 for the year 2021, of which (602,000 or 96%) will be in Africa. Worldwide, children under the age of five are the most vulnerable to malaria. They accounted for 80% of malaria-related deaths [8].

Like most countries in sub-Saharan Africa, malaria is the leading cause of mortality and morbidity in Mali [9].

In Mali, the malaria incidence rate in 2022 is 172 per 1000; according to the district health information software (DHIS2). A survey of knowledge, attitudes and practices is a representative study conducted among a given population to identify knowledge (K), attitudes (A) and practices (P) on a specific subject. It is a strategic tool for identifying the educational needs of a specific target group. It evolves around three points, namely the level of knowledge, the attitudes motivating the behaviour and the preventive and management practices of the target populations [10]. The aim of this qualitative analysis is to develop concepts that will enable us to understand phenomena and group behaviour in the fight against malaria. We also used a quantitative analysis to gather socio-demographic information, knowledge, attitudes and practices of the population; the aim of this quantitative analysis is to verify the extent to which the information and hypotheses can be generalised and to deduce statistically measurable conclusions.

While technical strategies are physical preventive measures, the knowledge, attitudes and practices of populations at risk can also play a role in preventing the disease. A study carried out in Ouéléssébougou on people's knowledge, attitudes, practices and malaria morbidity among pregnant women and children aged 0-5 years found that the population recognised the symptoms of malaria well. They turned first to the CsCom. This study also showed that malaria is still the leading public health problem, being the main cause of consultations at the health centre, and that mosquito nets were rarely used correctly [11]. In another study, this time carried out in Niamakoro (a peri-urban district of Bamako), it was found that people were able to recognise the symptoms and mode of transmission of malaria (mosquito bites were the most frequently mentioned by participants) and that mosquito nets were the most widely used means of

preventing malaria [12].
This knowledge can enable the populations concerned to adopt better attitudes and practices towards the disease, such as visiting health centres when the signs of malaria are known. It is with this in mind that the present study proposes to carry out a CAP study in the Baco-Djicoroni district.
The Baco-Djicoroni district is made up of 6 sectors. In two of the six sectors, namely ACI (Agence de Cession Immobilière) and Golf, the majority of the population has a medium to high income, while in the other 4 sectors (Hèrèmakono, Plateau, Dougoukoro and Sokoura) the majority of the population has a low income.
For various reasons, many families in these areas do not bring their patients to the community health centre. This could be explained by the fact that people do not have the necessary knowledge, attitudes and practices to deal with malaria, especially when it comes to prevention. Given the high rate of malaria consultations in the Baco-Djicoroni health area, it is important to investigate the levels of knowledge, practices and attitudes of the area's population with regard to preventive measures against the disease.
If this population is well informed about the usefulness of malaria prevention measures and if they practise these preventive measures correctly, this could considerably reduce the malaria transmission rate in this population.
Consequently, the hypothesis of this study is that the levels of knowledge, practices and attitudes of the populations of the Baco-Djicoroni health area do not contribute to malaria prevention.
The aim of this study is to assess the levels of knowledge, attitudes and practices of people in the Baco-Djicoroni health area regarding malaria prevention measures.

- Justification for the choice of study

It is important to study the behaviour, perception and/or attitude of individuals towards malaria. These are the factors that will determine the outcome of the disease: recovery, worsening, death. According to the WHO, the number of cases was 59 per 1,000 inhabitants exposed to the risk of malaria in 2020. In 2020, the number of deaths due to malaria was estimated at 15.3 per 100,000 exposed inhabitants [13]. The malaria prevalence rate in Mali is 19% [9].
Illness cruelly affects the body as well as other aspects of life. For this reason, it would be wise to study ways and means of prevention. In Mali, we can't talk about disease without looking at malaria, which is a major scourge. Such a disease is a threat to the country's development. This is all the more true because the periods of invalidity and premature death it causes greatly diminish the country's workforce. It therefore becomes imperative to consider the means

currently used to combat this scourge. Despite the many studies carried out on malaria in Mali, it is still rampant and continues to cause enormous damage. More than 54.4% of people still resort to self-medication to treat malaria without referring to a health professional [14].

With the specific aim of helping to reduce or halt the increase in new cases, it would be important to carry out an in-depth study at various levels of the social and economic sector into the knowledge, attitudes and practices of the population in relation to this scourge. The people of Baco-Djicoroni come from many different backgrounds.

So, in the fight against malaria, there is the possibility of curative treatment, which can give conclusive results. However, given the recurrent nature of the disease and the germ's current level of resistance to chemical products, preventive treatment would be the best solution. The aim of this study is to assess people's knowledge, attitudes and behavioural practices with regard to malaria prevention. To this end, the study focused on the inhabitants of our place of residence, Baco-Djicoroni.

Chapter 3

OBJECTIVES

3. Objectives

3.1.1 general objective

To assess knowledge, attitudes and practices relating to malaria prevention in the Baco-Djicoroni community.

3.1.2 specific objectives

- Describe the socio-demographic characteristics of the participants;
- Describe the Baco-Djicoroni community's level of knowledge about malaria prevention;
- Describe the attitudes and practices of the Baco-Djicoroni community with regard to malaria prevention;
- Identify the sources of information on malaria prevention in the Baco-Djicoroni community.

Chapter 4

THEORETICAL FRAMEWORK

4. Theoretical framework or conceptual approach

4.1 Definition of concepts

Malaria: is a fatal disease caused by a parasite of the genus *Plasmodium* transmitted by the bite of a female mosquito of the genus Anopheles, the "malaria vector". The disease is preventable and curable [6].

CAP: a CAP is a representative study conducted among a specific population to identify the knowledge (C), attitudes (A) and practices (P) of a population on a specific topic [10].

Knowledge: the fact or manner of knowing [15].

Attitude: way of behaving, behaviour that corresponds to a disposition [16].

Practice: voluntary activity aimed at achieving concrete results (as opposed to theory) [17]. **Health area**: a basic geographical unit containing a minimum population of five thousand (5,000) inhabitants and forming the area in which a community health centre is set up and operates; it is determined by consensus between the communities concerned [18].

Prevention: is the set of actions, attitudes and behaviours that aim to avoid the occurrence of disease or injury or to maintain and improve health [19].

4.2 Epidemiology of malaria

Malaria is by far the most important tropical parasitic disease in the world, claiming more victims than any other communicable disease except tuberculosis.

Malaria is by far the most important tropical parasitic disease in the world, claiming more lives than any other communicable disease in sub-Saharan Africa, accounting for more than 90% of all cases. Mortality from malaria is particularly high among children.

In many countries, malaria control programmes had been remarkably successful, but their abandonment in favour of primary health care and the emergence of insecticide resistance in mosquitoes led to a resurgence of the disease and new epidemics. In addition, chloroquine-resistant strains of *Plasmodium falciparum* have emerged.

The epidemiology of malaria depends on three factors:

- the presence of people with malaria, as humans are the only reservoir of malaria parasites

- the presence of insect vectors (anopheles) and water where the larvae develop
- an average temperature of 15°C or above, an essential factor for the sexual cycle of Anopheles parasites [20].

4.3 Malaria vector

The main malaria vectors in Mali are the *Anopheles gambiae s.l.* and *Anopheles funestus s.l.* complexes [21]. Anopheles is a genus of mosquitoes of the order Diptera, family Culicidae and subfamily Anophelinae [22]. Of the more than 500 known species of Anopheles, nearly fifty are capable of transmitting Plasmodium [23].

The distribution of anophelines around the world is much more extensive than that of malaria, hence the notion of "anophelism without malaria".

In Mali, members of the *An. gambiae s.l.* and *An. funestus* complex transmit malaria between 6pm and 6am. Their average lifespan is around one month. The level of infection can vary from one to one thousand infecting bites per person per year [24] (Figure 1).

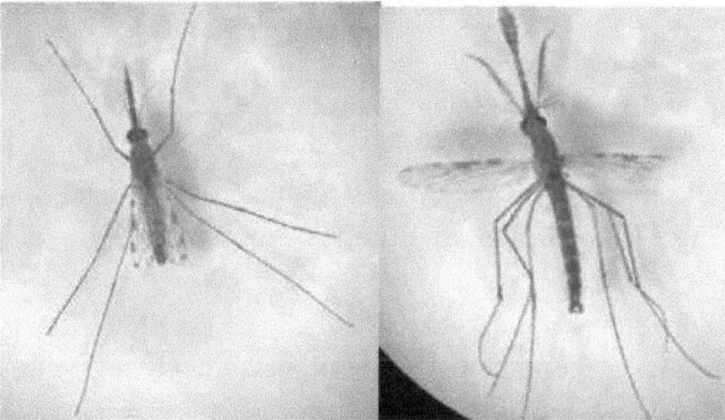

Figure 1 : Adult *An. gambiae s.l.* Female (left) and male (right)
(source: Vector genetics and genomics laboratory /MRTC)

4.4 Pathogen

Malaria is caused by a protozoan parasite, *Plasmodium*. There are many species of *Plasmodium* that infect various animal species, but only five are found in human pathology: *P. falciparum*, *P. malariae*, *P. ovale*, *P. vivax* and *P. knowlesi*. P. knowlesi usually parasitises signs (macaques) in South-East Asia and has recently been transmitted to humans[25].

- *Plasmodium falciparum* :

P. falciparum is the most widespread throughout the world, it develops more resistance to antimalarial drugs and is responsible for serious and potentially fatal clinical forms[26]. It is responsible for malignant third-grade fever. Ninety-five per cent (95%) of malaria cases worldwide are due to *P. falciparum*[25]. The incubation period is 7 to 15 days (often 10 to 12 days) [26]. It is responsible for 99% of malaria cases in Africa [24].

- *Plasmodium vivax* :

Responsible for benign third-grade fever, it is more widely distributed than *P. falciparum*, except in sub-Saharan Africa. It predominates in the Americas (64% of cases). It is not as harmless as some people think: severe, even fatal, forms have been reported in India and Amazonia [24]. The incubation period is 12 to 18 days [26]. Erythrocytic schizogony occurs every 48 hours. A third fever is observed. The latter is generally benign. However, there is a possibility of late relapses lasting three to five years [27].

- *Plasmodium ovale* :

It occurs in intertropical Africa and certain regions of the Pacific. Like *P. vivax*, which it closely resembles, it is responsible for benign third-grade fever [2]. It has an incubation period of 12 to 18 days [25]. It has a benign course but, as with *P. vivax*, late relapses (5 years) can be observed. Schematically, *P. ovale* is said to replace *P. vivax* where the latter species does not exist [2]. It is composed of 2 subspecies*: P. ovale curtisi and P. ovale wallikeri*, described in 2011 in Central Africa, and remains less dangerous than *P. falciparum* [28].

- *Plasmodium malariae* :

It occurs on all three continents (Africa, South-East Asia and South America), albeit much more sporadically. It differs from other species in a number of ways:

- Longer incubation period (15 to 21 days),
- A different fever periodicity (72-hour erythrocyte cycle responsible for quarte fever)
- And above all, its ability to cause very late relapses (up to 20 years after returning from the endemic zone). The physiological mechanisms responsible for these late relapses have not been fully elucidated. Some suggest the presence of latent merozoites in the lymphatic tract. The infection is benign, but *P. malariae* can sometimes lead to renal complications [2].

- *Plasmodium knowlesi* :

It occurs in forest areas of South-East Asia. It is morphologically similar to *P. malariae*. It differs from other species in that it has a 24-hour erythrocytic cycle, which causes a daily fever. There are rare severe, even fatal, forms with high parasitaemia. To date, no chemoresistance has been observed in this species [2]. The course is potentially serious and the infection must be treated in the same way as *P. falciparum* [24].

4.5. Epidemiology of malaria in Mali

Since 2016-2017, WHO technical guidelines have recommended using malaria risk stratification to better target the malaria control intervention.

Malaria risk stratification is defined as the classification of geographical areas according to epidemiological, entomological, environmental and socio-economic factors that determine susceptibility and vulnerability to malaria transmission. Each defined stratum is composed of health districts with similar malaria incidence patterns.

Malaria risk was stratified according to spatial heterogeneity of malaria incidence, prevalence of malaria in children under 5, distribution of vector resistance, access to health facilities, child mortality and seasonality of malaria transmission. The targeting of malaria control interventions was discussed with the National Malaria Control Programme and the various financial partners.

Between 2017-2019, the median incidence in the 75 health districts was 129.34 cases per 1,000 person-years (standard deviation=86.48) [29]. Risk stratification identified 12 health districts in the very low transmission zone, 19 in the low transmission zone, 20 in the moderate transmission zone and 24 in the high transmission zone. Poor access to health facilities and increased vector resistance to standard insecticides were observed in the high transmission zones.

Eight combinations of interventions were selected for implementation, using stratification, the presence of pyrethroid resistance in vectors, infant and child mortality, and the presence of vector resistance to standard insecticides.

and forecast financial resources.

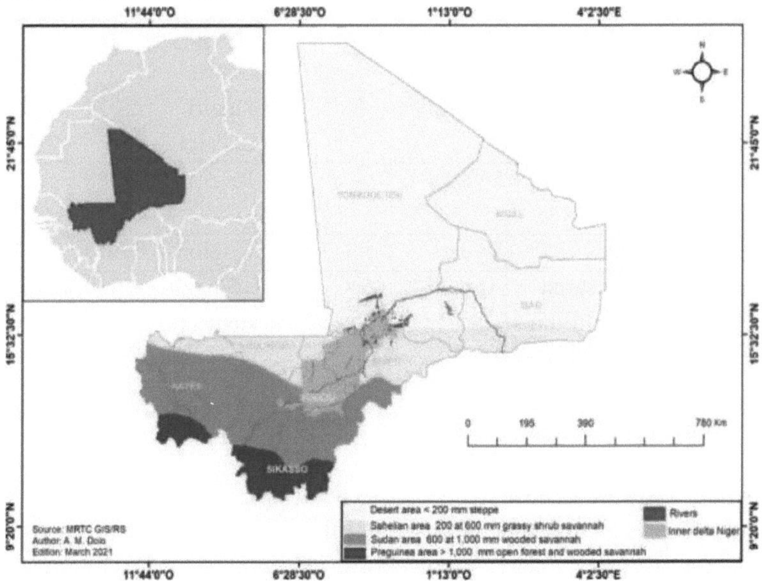

Figure 2: Mali's eco-climatic zones (Source: MRTC GIS/RS)

Mali is divided into 11 regions (including the District of Bamako) and 75 health districts. The healthcare system is organised according to a 3-level pyramid (health district level, regional level and national level) [30] .

Table I: Collection of variable data relating to malaria in entomology and the environment

Variables	Sources	Resolution/timing	Scale	Periods
Population	DHIS2	Annual	Health district	2017-2019
Casde malaria	DHIS2	Monthly	Health district	2017-2019
Access to care	DHIS2	Monthly	Health district	2017-2019
Rate visits to healthcare facilities** (in millions of euros)	DHIS2	Annual	Health district	2017-2019
Rainfall	IMERG v6	Monthly	Health district	2017-2019
Relative humidity	AIRS	Monthly	Health district	2017-2019
Temperature	MERRA - 2	Monthly	Health district	2017-2019
NDVI	MODIS Terra	Monthly	Health district	2017-2019
Prevalence of malaria	DHS	5 years	Region	2018
Infant mortality	DHS	5 years	Region	2018
Entomological data	Research institution s (Sentinel site)	Annual	15 health districts s	2010, 2015,2016 ,201 7 and 2019

NDVI: Normalized Difference Vegetation Index, DHIS2: District Health

Information Software 2, IMERG: Integrated Multisatellite Retrievals for GPM, AIRS: Atmospheric Infrared Sounder, MERRA-2: Modern-Era Retrospective analysis for Research and Applications, Version 2, MODIS: Moderate

Resolution Imaging Spectroradiometer, DHS: Demographic and Health Survey, Research institutions: Malaria Research and Training Center (MRTC), Laboratory of
Applied Molecular Biology (LBMA), and National Institute of Public Health (INSP),
Sentinel sites: Koulikoro (Tienfala), Kati (Dandoly), Kankass (Socoura), Djenné (Madiama), Mopti (Tongorongo), Tominian (Ouena), Bamako, Bla, Sikasso, Bougouni, Selingue, Niono, Kayes, and Kita.

1 Access to healthcare facilities is the proportion of the population living within 5 km of a healthcare facility.

2 * The attendance rate at health facilities is the ratio of new consultations to the total population x 100.

3 ** Mortality among children aged between 6 and 59 months for the period 2012-2017 according to the EDS 2018.

[29]

Data on malaria, entomology and the environment were obtained from the local health information system, the 2018 Demographic and Health Survey (DHS), the National Aeronautics and Space Administration and Malian research institutions working on malaria (Table I).

4.6.The biological cycle of malaria

When taking a blood meal, the female Anopheles injects infecting sporozoites contained in its salivary glands into the bloodstream through the puncture site. The sporozoites reach the hepatocytes in less than half an hour after inoculation, where they multiply to form liver schizonts known as "blue bodies". These schizonts burst and release the merozoites into the bloodstream, where they actively penetrate the erythrocytes. This first phase corresponds to exo-erythrocytic schizogony. In the red blood cells, the merozoites become trophozoites, then schizonts (rosettes) which burst and destroy the red blood cells to release second-generation merozoites which can infect other red blood cells: this is endo-erythrocytic schizogony (which corresponds to the phase of clinical manifestations). At the end of the endo-erythrocytic cycle, certain trophozoites transform into parasitic elements with sexual potential: male and female gametocytes. During a blood meal, the mosquito ingests the gametocytes which, by ex-flagellation of the males, give the microgametes (male gametes) and by expulsion of the chromatic corpuscle of the females give the macrogametes (female gametes). The fusion of a male gamete and a female gamete produces a mobile egg with 2n chromosomes (the only diploid element), the ookinete. The ookinete passes through the wall of the Anopheles stomach and attaches itself to the outside of the stomach to become an oocyst from which the sporozoites (n chromosomes) develop. The oocyst bursts and releases the sporozoites, which migrate into the salivary glands of the Anopheles, from where they are inoculated into the human during a new blood meal.

The cycle occurs successively in humans and in Anopheles [31] (Figure 3).

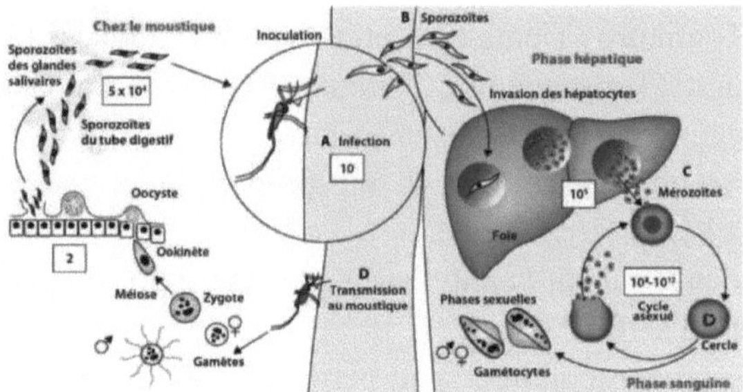

Figure 3: Life cycle of the malaria parasite (Source: https ://www.google.com/sciencedirect.com)

4.7.Overview of malaria

4.7.1. Transmission

The malaria parasite is transmitted by female Anopheles mosquitoes, which bite mainly between dusk and dawn. Transmission can rarely occur through the blood, by transfusion, following a blood exposure accident (BSE) or by injection when drug users share injection equipment. There is a risk of blood transmission only from fresh blood with intact red blood cells. Maternal-foetal transmission is rare.

4.7.2. Incubation

The incubation period between the anopheles bite and the first clinical signs depends on the species involved: 7 to 15 days (often 10 to 12 days) for *P. falciparum*, 12 to 18 days for *P. vivax* and *P. ovale* and 10 to 15 days for *P. knowlesi*. The incubation period for *P. falciparum* may be prolonged if the patient has been on chemoprophylaxis or has partial immunity.

4.7.3. Contagious period

The mosquito becomes infectious 2 weeks after ingesting the plasmodium and remains so for life (lifespan of around 1 month). The patient's blood is contaminated when gametocytes are present in the circulation, i.e. from the 4^{e} day of symptoms for *P. ovale* and *P. vivax* and from the 15^{e} day for *P. falciparum* and *P. malariae*. Gametocytes remain in the blood for several weeks, despite treatment. Their presence does not indicate active infection.

4.7.4. Symptom

Any fever in a patient returning from a malaria-endemic area (7 days to three months, rarely longer) should be considered diagnostic of malaria ("any fever in a patient returning from a malaria-endemic area is **malaria** until proven otherwise"). The clinical manifestations of malaria vary greatly in expression and severity, and depend on both the plasmodial species and its host [26].

4.7.5. Clinical signs of malaria

- Simple malaria

This clinical form corresponds to the description of the classic triad of malaria attacks: "chills, heat, sweating" occurring every 2 or 3 days. In practice, it is only typically observed in *P. vivax, P. ovale and P. malariae* infestations.

The attack usually begins in the evening and lasts about ten hours, successively associating :

- Shivering stage: agitated by violent shivering, the patient huddles under their sheets while their temperature rises to 39°C. The spleen enlarges and blood pressure falls. This phase lasts about an hour.
- Heat stage: the temperature may exceed 40°C, the skin is dry and burning and the patient throws off their sheets. This phase is accompanied by headaches and abdominal pain, and lasts 3 to 4 hours. The spleen diminishes in volume.
- Sweating stage: the patient sweats profusely. The patient emits dark urine, and the temperature suddenly plummets, sometimes even going into hypothermia. Blood pressure rises again. This stage lasts 2 to 4 hours and is accompanied by a feeling of well-being and euphoria, bringing the attack to a close [32].
- Severe malaria

Severe malaria is characterised by biological confirmation (positive RDT or GE/FM) with the presence of *P. falciparum* associated with one or more of the following clinical and/or biological manifestations: **Clinical manifestations**

The most relevant events to take into account for better management are the following**:**

- prostration: as a rule, extreme weakness (unable to walk or sit up);
- disturbed consciousness or coma: Glasgow score < 10; Blantyre ≤ 2 ;
- respiratory distress (acidosis);
- Repeated convulsions: at least two per 24 hours;
- Cardiovascular collapse or shock (systolic BP < 70 mm Hg in adults and 50 mm Hg in children);
- pulmonary oedema (radiological); abnormalities specified in children ;
- abnormal bleeding (coagulation disorder) purely clinical definition - jaundice: clinical or total bilirubin > 50 μmol/l ;
- macroscopic haemoglobinuria (coca cola or dark-coloured urine).

Biological manifestations

The biological disturbances observed are as follows:

- severe anaemia or extreme pallor: Hb < 5 g/dl or Ht < 15% ;
- hypoglycaemia: blood glucose < 2.2 mmol/l or 0.4 g/l ;
- metabolic acidosis: PH < 7.35 or bicarbonate < 15 mmol/l ;
- hyperlactataemia: plasma lactates > 5 mmol/l;
- hyperparasitaemia: parasitaemia ≥ 4% in non-immune subjects;
- renal failure: creatinine > 265 μmol/l [33].

4.8.Diagnosis of malaria

4.8.1. Biological diagnosis

In the laboratory, the diagnosis is based on the detection and identification of the parasite by direct microscopic examination after staining a thick drop or blood smear.

- **Thick drop :**

It is used to identify the malaria parasite and quantify parasitaemia. A drop of blood is placed on a glass slide up to $1cm^2$, then dried for a long time, and finally the red blood cells are dehaemoglobinised and stained with May- Grün Wald-Giemsa. The reading is taken under the microscope [34].

- **Blood smear :**

This is a rapid test that calculates the percentage of red blood cells parasitised and identifies the plasmodial species responsible for the disease.

NB: tests for haematozoa should be carried out before any chemotherapy is started.

4.8.2. Serological diagnosis

Over the last twenty years, a great deal of work has gone into malaria serodiagnosis, leading to the development of tried and tested methods and reagents. To be precise, this serodiagnosis must be carried out under very strict technical conditions. In the end, these conditions are limited and, on the whole, only apply to cases where parasitological diagnosis is impossible. Finally, interpretation of the results depends on the method and reagents used. Serological reactions include indirect immunofluorescence, indirect haemagglutination, ELISA and immunodiffusion [35].

4.9 National guidelines for the treatment of malaria

Simple malaria can be effectively treated orally. The most effective treatments today are Artemisinin-based Combination Therapies (ACTs). They are effective in treating uncomplicated malaria within 3 days.

Severe malaria can be treated with :

- artesunate injection,
- artemether injection,
- quinine injection.

Switch to the oral route as soon as the patient's condition permits

4.9.1. Simple malaria

CsCom, CSref, hospitals and other health facilities:

The treatment of uncomplicated malaria in children under 5, adolescents and adults is based on three elements:

- **specific treatment**: based specifically on the fixed combinations Artemether + Lumefantrine or Artesunate + Amodiaquine
- **Adjuvant treatment**: based on medication, i.e. paracetamol, iron and folic acid if anaemia.
- **advice for patients**

a. Specific treatment

Table II: Collection of variable data relating to malaria in entomology and the environment

Age/weight groups	Day 1		Day 2		Day 3	
	morning	evening	morning	evening	morning	evening
05 - 14 kg (2 months to 3 years)	1cp	1cp	1cp	1cp	1cp	1cp
15 - 24 kg (4 years to 6 years)	2cp	2cp	2cp	2cp	2cp	2cp
25 - 34 kg (7 to 10 years)	3cp	3cp	3cp	3cp	3cp	3cp
≥ 35 kg and adults	4cp	4cp	4cp	4cp	4cp	4cp

Source: https://www. severemalaria. org/sites/mmv-

smo/files/content/attachments/2017-07-25/Mali%20treatment%20 guidelines 0. pdf .

Table III: Presentation and dosage of artesunate-amodiaquine

Intervalde weight (approximate age range)	Presentation	1er treatment day	2e treatment day	3e treatment day
≥4 .5 kg to <9kg (2 to 11 months)	25mg/67.5mg blister pack of 3cp	1tablet	1tablet	1tablet
≥ 9kg to <18kg (1 to 11 years)	50mg /135mg blister pack of 3cp	1tablet	1tablet	1tablet
≥ 18kg to < 36kg (6 to 13 years)	100mg /2703m g blister pack of 3cp	1tablet	1tablet	1 tablet
≥ 36kg (14 years	100mg/270mg	2 tablets	2 tablets	2 tablets

and over)	blister pack of 6cp			

Source: https://www. severemalaria. org/sites/mmv-

smo/files/content/attachments/2017-07-25/Mali%20treatment%20 guidelines 0. pdf .

NB: The first dose must be taken under supervision. If the child vomits within 30 minutes, repeat the dose.

Action to be taken :

If signs persist, it is important to re-examine the patient and repeat the biological diagnosis.

If the patient has followed the treatment correctly and the biological test is negative:

- look for other causes of fever or refer for assessment.

If the treatment is not followed :

- resume treatment under medical supervision.

If laboratory tests are not possible:

- refer to a higher level.

b. Adjuvant treatment

The medicines and dosage to be administered are :

- paracetamol 500 mg; 15 to 20 mg/kg every 6 hours ;
- iron 200 mg: 2 tablets/day (adult) or 10 mg/kg/day (child) if anaemia ;
- folic acid 5 mg: 1 tablet/day if anaemia.

c. Advice for patients

When should you return immediately?

- if fever persists ;
- if the child has difficulty drinking and is unable to eat;
- if convulsion (eye twitching) ;
- if unable to sit ;
- if vomiting persists ;
- if it becomes unconscious ;
- if pallor or jaundice ;
- if there is blood in the stools;
- if dark urine ;
- if breathing difficulty.

Focus on :

- Follow-up visit after 3 days of treatment if the problem persists;
- the need to continue feeding and increase fluids;
- Continue to take the medicine even if the patient feels better;

- malaria prevention (use of insecticide-treated mosquito nets for children and pregnant women, IPT for pregnant women and CPS for children aged between 3 and 59 months);
- early recourse to the Cscom for subsequent episodes.

4.9.2. Severe malaria

At CsCom/Csref/hospital level

The treatment of severe and complicated malaria in children under 5 years of age, pregnant women, adolescents and adults is based on two elements:

- **emergency treatment of complications:** vital for the patient. Death may be caused by **the disease itself or by its complications**.
- **specific antimalarial treatment:** this is essential and extremely urgent, and must be administered very quickly to halt the progress of the disease.

a. Emergency treatment of complications

Symptomatic treatment is used to correct hypoglycaemia, dehydration and anaemia, reduce fever, stop convulsions and manage coma and respiratory, renal and cardiovascular problems.

- **Treatment of hypoglycaemia :**

In children and adolescents, administer slowly by IV:

- 3 to 5 ml for 10% glucose serum where
- 1 ml/kg for 30% glucose serum.

For adults, administer slowly by IV:

- 3 to 5 ml/kg for 10% glucose serum where
- 1 ml/kg for 30% glucose serum where
- 25 ml of 50% serum glucose: if you only have 50% serum glucose, dilute it.

one volume in 4 volumes of sterile water to obtain a 10% solution (for example, 0.4ml/kg of 50% glucose with 1.6ml/kg of water for injection or 4ml of 50% glucose with 16ml of water for injection). Hypertonic glucose (> 20%) is not recommended as it has an irritant effect on peripheral veins.

If intravenous administration is not possible, give glucose or another sugar solution through a nasogastric tube.

- **Treatment of dehydration :**
- Administer 100 ml/kg of Ringer's solution over 2 or 4 hours,
- Reassess the patient afterwards to determine water requirements and the state of dehydration.
- **Treatment of convulsions :**
- Administer diazepam at a dose of 0.5 mg/kg intra rectally (IR) or IM;
- If convulsions persist, 10 to 15 mg/kg parenteral phenobarbital.

- **Treatment of anaemia :**

If severe anaemia (haemoglobin < 5 g/dl) :

Administer blood as a matter of urgency: 20ml/kg of whole blood for 4 hours with furosemide or 10ml/kg of packed red blood cells in children. If **transfusion is not possible:**

- Carry out pre-transfer treatment before sending the patient to a centre with a blood transfusion service.

- **In case of coma :**
- Assess the stage of coma (Blantyre or Glasgow scale),
- Place the patient in the lateral position,
- Aspirate secretions and clear the airways,
- Insert a nasogastric feeding tube,
- Take a venous line,
- Place a urinary catheter,
- Change the patient's position every 4 hours,
- Measure urine volume (diuresis).

- **In the event of breathing difficulties: (Acute lung oedema)**
- Put the patient in a semi-seated position, administer oxygen and furosemide IV: 2 to 4 mg/kg;
- If possible, evacuate the patient to an intensive care unit.

- **In case of renal insufficiency :**
- Administer fluids if the patient is dehydrated: 20 ml/kg of isotonic saline, 1 to 2 mg/kg of furosemide.
- Placing a bladder catheter

If the patient does not pass urine within 24 hours :

- Transfer to a centre for dialysis.

b. Specific antimalarial treatment

The drugs recommended for the treatment of severe malaria are: artesunate, artemether or quinine. **Artesunate** is the drug of choice for the treatment of severe malaria. It can be administered by intravenous (IV) or intramuscular (IM) injection.

✓ **Artesunate**

2.4 mg/kg of body weight administered intravenously (IV) or intramuscularly (IM) on admission (t= 0), then 12h and 24h later and thereafter once daily for patients weighing 20 kg or more until the patient is able to take oral medication.

For children weighing less than 20 kg: Artesunate 3 mg/kg body weight according to the times indicated above.

If injectable artesunate is not available, it can be replaced by artemether or

quinine:
Take over with oral CTA as soon as the patient can swallow.

✓ **Artemether**

Dosage and administration :
Intramuscular treatment over 5 days: the dose is 3.2 mg/kg body weight in one injection on admission, followed by 1.6 mg/kg in one injection per day for 4 days.

Table IV: dosage and administration of artemether in children aged 0-5 years: 20 mg ampoules.

Age	Weight	Day 1	Day 2	Day 3	Day 4	Day 5
>1 year	5 - 9 kg	1 ampoule	½ bulb	½ bulb	½ bulb	½ bulb
2 - 5 years	10 - 15 kg	2 bulbs	1 ampoule	1 ampoule	1 ampoule	1 ampoule

Source: https://www. severemalaria. org/sites/mmv-smo/files/content/attachments/2017-07- 25/Mali%20treatment%20 guidelines 0. pdf .

Table V: dosage and administration of artemether in subjects over 5 years of age: 80 mg ampoules.

Age	Weight	Day 1	Day 2	Day 3	Day 4	Day 5
6 - 13 years	16 - 35 kg	1 ampoule	½ bulb	½ bulb	½ bulb	½ bulb
14 years and over	≥ 35 kg	2 bulbs	1 ampoule	1 ampoule	1 ampoule	1 ampoule

Source: https://www. severemalaria. org/sites/mmv-smo/files/content/attachments/2017-07- 25/Mali%20treatment%20 guidelines 0. pdf .

Take over with oral CTAs as soon as the patient can swallow.

✓ **Quinine**

There are two methods of injecting quinine: quinine administered by intravenous infusion and quinine administered intramuscularly.
Recommended dosage :
- Quinine administered by intravenous infusion :
Loading dose: 20 mg quinine salt kg on admission in adults and children.
NB: the loading dose is only administered when the patient has not taken quinine in the previous 24 hours or Mefloquine in the previous 7 days,

otherwise the maintenance dose is used.
Maintenance dose :
Children :
Dosage: 10 mg/kg of quinine hydrochloride salts (8.3 mg base) diluted in 10 ml/kg of 10% glucose serum (or 4.3% dextrose or 0.9% saline for diabetics).
Duration of infusion: 2 - 4 hours
Interval between infusions: 8 hours
Switch to the oral route with CTA as soon as the patient can swallow
Where
Dosage: 15 mg/kg of quinine hydrochloride salts (12.4 mg base) diluted in 10 ml/kg of 10% glucose serum (or 4.3% dextrose or 0.9% saline for diabetics).
Duration of infusion: 2 - 4 hours
Interval between infusions: 12 hours
Switch to the oral route with CTAs as soon as the patient can swallow.
Adults :
10 mg/kg of quinine salts (8.3 mg base) diluted in 10 ml/kg of a hypertonic solution infused over 4 hours with 10% glucose, 4.3% dextrose or (0.9% isotonic saline for diabetics).
Interval between infusions: 8 hours,
Duration of infusion: 4 hours.
The duration of treatment with quinine is seven (7) days.
NB: take quinine tablets with water to prevent hypoglycaemia.
- Intramuscular quinine :
If administration by intravenous (IV) infusion is not possible, give the same dose (10 mg/kg) intra-muscularly (IM) every 8 hours and continue until the patient is able to take the treatment orally. The injection should be made into the antero-external aspect of the thigh.
Give the patient sugar water to prevent hypoglycaemia [33].

4.9.3. Treatment of malaria in pregnant women

a. Simple malaria

- first trimester of pregnancy: quinine tablets at a dose of 10 mg/kg every 8 hours for 7 days.
- second and third trimesters of pregnancy: CTA [Artemether + Lumefantrine(ALU) or Artesunate + Amodiaquine (ASAQ)].

b. Severe malaria

Pregnant women suffering from severe malaria should be given parenteral antimalarial drugs without delay, regardless of the stage of pregnancy and without reducing the dose. The mortality rate due to severe malaria during pregnancy is around 50%, which is higher than in non-pregnant women.

Artesunate is the treatment of choice. If this drug is not available, artemether is preferable to quinine at the end of pregnancy, as quinine is associated with a 50% risk of hypoglycaemia.
Switch to the oral route as soon as the patient can swallow (compressed quinine for pregnant women in the first trimester of pregnancy and CTA from the second trimester of pregnancy) [36].

4.10. Malaria prevention

Malaria prevention is based on antimalarial chemoprophylaxis and vector control.

4.10.1. Chemoprevention of malaria

Chemoprevention of malaria concerns the most vulnerable groups: pregnant women, newborns and children.

a. Pregnant women

Sulfadoxine + pyrimethamine: comes in tablets containing 500 mg of sulfadoxine and 25 mg of pyrimethamine; dosage: 3 tablets taken as a single dose (adults). In Mali, it is used as part of the intermittent preventive treatment (IPT) of malaria in pregnant women recommended by the PNLP from the 2nd[e] trimester of pregnancy.

b. New topics

Chemoprophylaxis refers to the administration of infra-therapeutic doses of antimalarial drugs at sufficiently regular intervals to prevent malaria. This treatment should be given to subjects exposed to a high risk of malaria. The choice of chemoprophylaxis should be discussed and adapted to each traveller. It depends on the area visited (intensity of transmission and level of resistance to antimalarial drugs), the season and the individual concerned (age, pregnant woman, lifestyle, etc.). There are 3 groups:

> Groupel : zone without chloroquinoresistance: this group covers mainly Central American countries, Haiti and the Dominican Republic. > Group 2: Isolated chloroquine resistance zone: Part of India and Sri Lanka are concerned.

> Group 3: areas of high prevalence of chloroquine resistance and multi-drug resistance. The number of countries in this group is constantly increasing. It now includes all the countries of sub-Saharan Africa, in particular Mali [2].

c. The children

This chemoprophylaxis concerns both children living in non-endemic areas and children under 5 in malaria-endemic areas. In endemic zones with periods of high transmission, according to recent WHO recommendations, all children under the age of 5 should receive a curative dose of antimalarial drugs during the period of high transmission. This is known as chemoprevention of seasonal malaria (CPS).

4.10.2. Vector control

Vector control is one of the essential malaria control strategies advocated in Mali. Its aim is to reduce or even eliminate malaria transmission. Its main components are :

- Larvae control,
- Reducing human-vector contact (use of insecticide-impregnated materials, spraying inside and outside the home).
- The same guidelines apply to imported or locally manufactured mosquito nets and netting fabrics.

a. Fighting larvae

Communication activities and measures to prevent the proliferation of larval breeding sites must accompany development and urbanisation work.

b. Hygiene and sanitation

This approach must be taken into account at the level of decentralised authorities through the application of environmental health standards.

c. Combating malaria epidemics

Malaria epidemics are managed in accordance with Integrated Disease Surveillance and Response (IDSR) guidelines. During epidemics, malaria cases are managed using ACTs for uncomplicated cases and quinine for severe cases. Interruption of transmission recommends widespread indoor residual spraying in epidemic areas [37].

Chapter 5

METHODOLOGICAL APPROACH

5. Methodological approach

5.1.Type and period of study

This is a descriptive cross-sectional study. It ran from June to November 2021.

5.2.Choice and description of the study framework

This study took place throughout the community covered by the Baco-Djicoroni ASACO.

5.2.1. Place of study

Baco-Djicoroni is a district of Bamako located in Commune V. It is located on the right bank of the River Niger and borders the districts of Kalaban-Coro to the south-west, Torokorobougou to the north-east, Sabalibougou to the east and the River Niger or Djoliba to the north-west.

Baco-Djicoroni was the former hunting reserve of the Diakité, who crossed the River Niger every day in dug-out canoes to hunt down animals, hence the name Baco-Djicoroni, "Djicoroni" meaning river and "Baco" meaning the other side. For a long time, this district was a gigantic field of mango trees, where hunting and cultivation went hand in hand, and where the winding dirt roads were no wider than the footsteps of pedestrians. These mango trees are now disappearing due to the recent and accelerated urbanisation of the district [38](Figure 4).

Baco-Djicoroni is divided into six sectors:

- sector 1: Dougoukoro, or the old village, which is the local people's neighbourhood.

and the first residents.

- sector 2: Sokoura is where the new arrivals have settled.
- sector 3: ACI (Agence de Cession Immobilière) south, because the ACI has developed it, is

commonly known as the ACI

- sector 4: ACI Est, commonly known as the Golf course
- sector 5: Le Plateau
- sector 6: Hèrèmakono (waiting for happiness in Bamanankan).

The population of Baco-Djicoroni was estimated at 148,589 in 2017, made up of

Bambara, Malinké, Soninké, Bwa, Peulh, Sonrhaï, Khassonké, Bozo, Dogon and others.
The most widely spoken language is Bamanankan. The religions practised are Islam, Christianity and Animism.
In terms of hydrography, Baco-Djicoroni is watered by the River Niger, or Djoliba in Bambara, which plays a major role in a number of economic activities, including gardening and fishing. The population engages in a variety of activities, the main one being trading.

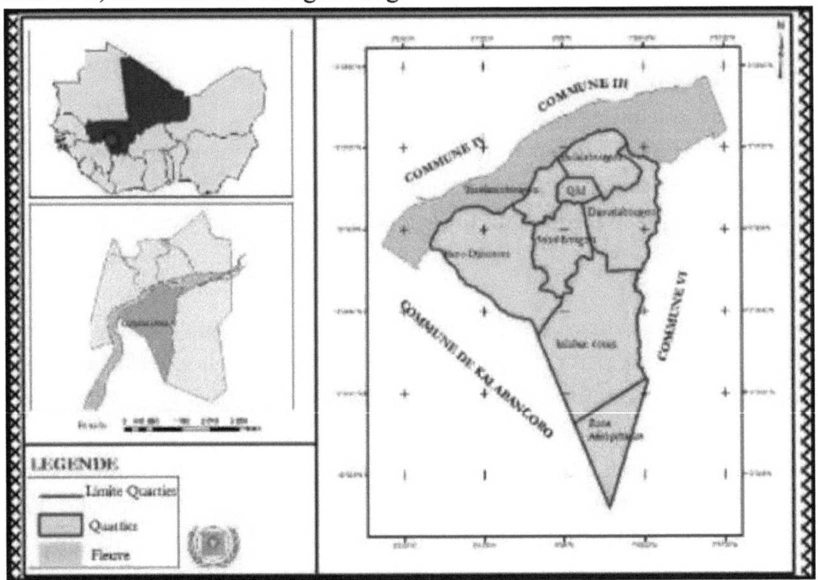

Figure 4: Map of Baco-Djicoroni (Source : *https://journals.openedition.org/eps/docannexe/image/7707/img-9-small580.png visited on 04/03/2021)*

5.2.2. Baco-Djicoroni health centre

The Baco-Djicoroni community health centre opened its doors on 1er January 1993. It occupies the premises of the former maternal and child health centre (PMI), which had already been built by the people of Baco-Djicoroni in the 1980s, but was only operational in 1992 due to a lack of staff and equipment.
It is the care unit created by the Baco-Djicoroni community health association (AScom Baco Dji), a not-for-profit association set up in October 1992 under receipt No. 1251 MECATS-DNAT.
In addition to its community nature, the originality of AScom Baco-Dji lies in six (6) principles:

- Its self-financing and self-management through cost recovery, the sale of medicines and membership fees;

- the quality of the services offered and the welcome ;
- offering the full range of PMA services (minimum activity package);
- the provision of services at costs that are acceptable and accessible to local residents;
- achieving effective and sustainable results in the fight against the disease, reduction in morbidity and mortality among children and pregnant women;
- its geographical accessibility.

The main objective of AScom-Baco-Dji, through the services offered by the CsCom, is to contribute to improving the health of the entire population of the district through active and voluntary participation.

The CsCom is headed by a medical director and has a 22-strong technical staff, all of Malian nationality.

a) Organisational plan for the health centre

The CsCom comprises the following units:

- two dispensary units ;
- INN drug depot (Pharmacy) ;
- a biomedical analysis laboratory unit;
- an ultrasound unit.
- a nursing care unit.
- a maternity unit comprising :
  - an antenatal clinic;
  - a delivery room (with two delivery tables);
  - a post-delivery observation room;
  - a short-term hospitalisation room or infusion room containing around ten beds.
- an accounting and management office.

The medical director's accommodation is on the first floor.

The centre has a water and electricity supply.

The staff consists of :

- three GPs,
- a senior laboratory technician,
- a laboratory technician,
- three public health nurses,
- a state nurse,
- six midwives,
- two obstetric nurses,
- a matron, an accountant,
- an assistant accountant,
- a labourer and

- a caretaker.

b) Health centre operating plan

The centre is open to all patients who have purchased a consultation ticket, whether or not they are members.

Home

Patients are welcomed by the accountant, who then refers them to the appropriate units as required.

At consultation unit level

Adults (male or female) are referred directly to the CUR (curative) unit with their consultation ticket and arrival number.

Children are also referred to the outpatient department, after a number of vital signs have been taken (weight, height, weight/height ratio, temperature). The patient is examined and, once a diagnosis has been made, is given a prescription and, if necessary, an additional examination. In this case, the patient is referred to the laboratory.

At nursing unit level

Patients who come for nursing care are directed to the treatment room.

NB: Consultation tickets issued to members cost CFA300 for adults and CFA200 for children aged 0-14.

Non-members pay 750 CFA francs for adults and 600 CFA francs for children aged 0-14.

At laboratory level

This is a first-level laboratory, which carries out analyses, the main ones being: GE (thick drop), glycaemia, Widal and Félix serology, rhesus grouping, albumin and sugar tests in urine.

Pharmacy

The pharmacy only dispenses generic medicines in INN (International Non-proprietary Name) form, which are on the official list of essential medicines in Mali. Medicines are only dispensed on presentation of a prescription from the centre. External prescriptions are not dispensed.

Maternity ward:

- **Prenatal consultation**

The reception staff (Obstetric Nurse) issues the woman with a prenatal consultation and vaccination booklet, takes her details and then refers her to one of the midwives for the prenatal consultation.

- **Giving birth**

Women who come for a delivery are dealt with directly (they are immediately directed to the delivery room).

- **Postnatal consultations and family planning**

These are carried out by the midwives on a rota basis. The midwives also deal with birth registrations.

- **Information, education and communication (IEC)**

The IEC is carried out every day before consultations in the presence of all the midwives and matrons.

- **Preventive consultation for healthy children (CPES)**

The CPES is the service which is carried out after taking a consultation booklet, is also provided by the midwives, and any child presenting a particular pathology is immediately referred to the CUR (curative) level. It consists mainly of taking the child's weight, height, temperature and growth curve, checking vaccinations and hygiene, and giving advice to mothers.

- **Vaccination**

Takes place every Tuesday and Thursday at the centre, exclusively as a fixed strategy, and covers all the diseases targeted by the national vaccination programme. It is carried out after a vaccination certificate has been obtained.

At the CREN (Centre for Nutritional Recovery and Education), consultations are also held on Tuesdays and Thursdays in the hangar, which serves as both a weighing room and a women's education centre. Nutritional recovery concerns all children with a P/T index of less than 85%. It is an activity that is currently integrated into vaccination in order to reach as many women and children as possible through nutritional education. I.E.C. (information, education and communication) on nutrition is carried out before the start of activities.

Accounting and management

It is managed by an accountant. The various rates are set by the management committee. All receipts are paid to the accountant at the end of the day. The receipts collected by the accountant are paid to the management committee's treasurer, who in turn transfers them to the bank, where a receipt for payment is issued for justification purposes. The centre pays for itself entirely from the income generated by the various services offered and the sale of ME (essential medicine). Rigorous management of resources is ensured by the ASACO management committee, which reports on its activities to the Administrative Board every 3 months.

Administrative and technical management of the centre

This is the responsibility of the Medical Director, who reports regularly to the Management Committee. The department is divided into different units, each headed by a unit manager who reports regularly to the Medical Director.

Every fortnight, there is a meeting of all the staff to discuss the running and various problems of the centre.

5.3.Study population

The study covered residents of the Baco-Djicoroni neighbourhood aged 18 and over.

5.3.1. Inclusion criteria

Any adult (≥ 18 years old) living in Baco-Djicoroni selected for the study and having agreed to take part in the study.

5.3.2. Non-inclusion criteria

All residents of Baco-Djicoroni who have not given their consent for the study and/or are under 18 years of age.

5.3.3. Exclusion criteria

Any person was excluded from the study:

- Who expressed the wish to retire from the study at some point.
- Who did not fill in his questionnaire correctly.

5.3.4. Sampling

The sampling technique was random, with a simple selection of Baco-Djicoroni residents aged 18 and over.

The SurveyMonkey formula was used:

$$n = \frac{\frac{Z^2 p(1-p)}{e^2}}{1 + (\frac{Z^2 p(1-p)}{e^2 N})}$$

- N = population size,
- Z = confidence interval (z-score),
- e = margin of error (in decimal form),
- p = percentage value (in decimal form)[39].

For the year 2017, the population of Baco-Djicoroni is estimated at approximately 148,589 inhabitants, who constitute the study frame. On the basis that 50% of this population have prerequisites in terms of malaria prevention, with a confidence level of 95% for a margin of error of 5%, a minimum sample of 600 inhabitants was obtained.

Assuming that 80% of the people contacted will take part in the study, our sample size will therefore be 660 people.

The sample size to be considered is = 660 divided into 110 for each sector.

Operational definition

- **Anyone with a good knowledge of malaria**: anyone who can name fever as a sign of malaria, name mosquito bites as a cause of malaria, name the fact that sleeping under an insecticide-treated mosquito net helps protect against malaria.
- **Standard of living:** The standard of living is the way of life according to the

average income in a country [40].

The standard of living corresponds to what Eurostat calls "equivalised disposable income".

Consumption units are generally calculated using the modified OECD equivalence scale, which assigns 1 CU to the first adult in the household, 0.5 CU to other persons aged 14 or over and 0.3 CU to children under 14 [41].

- **Income:** what accrues to someone as remuneration for work or as the fruit of capital [42].

The average monthly per capita income in Mali is $73 (45,279.02 CFA francs), or $870 (539,626.72 CFA francs) per person per year. The average wage in Mali is €102.25 (67,029.70 Fcfa). This figure is based on the average salaries reported by Internet users living in the country [43].

- **Low income: a** family unit with an income below the threshold estimated on the basis of its size and the degree of urbanisation of the region in which it lives [44].
- **Average income:** This is the arithmetic mean of income for a given group of households or individuals [45]. It is also the dollar amount obtained by dividing the total income of all members of families (census/economic), persons aged 15 and over excluding families, or households by the number of families, non-family persons aged 15 and over, or households [46].
- **High income:** an increase in average per capita income.

5.4.Study schedule

Activities ^Periods	Nov -20	Dec -20	Janv -21	May -21	Sept - 21	Nov -21	May -22	April -23	July -23
Bibliographical research									
Drafting and validation of the protocol									
Collection of qualitative data									
Quantitative data collection									
Data entry, analysis and processing									
Writing a thesis									
Correction									

Final presentation of the document									

5.5.Survey techniques and tools

5.5.1. Quantitative data collection and analysis: questionnaire

This involved using a survey form during the study (survey form in appendix) and interviewing men and women (≥ 18 years old) living in the locality. The interview was directed, focusing on the socio-demographic information of the men and women; their knowledge of malaria, its transmission and prevention; their attitudes towards malaria and its prevention; and their malaria prevention practices.

The participants were asked to complete a questionnaire and the answers were recorded on a survey sheet drawn up for this purpose (questionnaire in appendices).

5.5.2. Qualitative data collection and analysis: focus group interview guide

With regard to the interview guide, the focus groups, with the permission of the interview participants, were recorded on a Dictaphone and translated into French for the purposes of analysis. The focus group interviews involved three (3) focus groups, each made up of six (6) people aged eighteen (18) or over. The responses were recorded using a Dictaphone for later analysis. The aim of this focus group study was to gain a better understanding of people's knowledge, attitudes and practices with regard to malaria prevention and treatment. The focus group was organised as follows:

- a group of six (6) men
- a group of six (6) women
- a mixed group of three (3) men and three (3) women.

5.6 Data entry and processing

The data collected on the survey form were carefully kept in a secure place by the interviewer until the end of the survey and were gradually entered into the Epi-info7 software. No identifiers were included.

The text was processed using Office Word 2010.

Epi info software was used to analyse the quantitative data.

The qualitative data recorded on a mobile phone was done via a dictaphone. The moderator was the translator and decipherer of what each member of the focus group had to say.

The content of the group discussions was translated into French and summarised by the moderator, in order to draw out the key substances.

5.7 Ethical considerations

Certified dual training in research ethics and in the Bamanankan language was provided in order to develop communication skills focused primarily on the language skills of the participants, and to provide better advice on compliance with the rules and ethical principles protecting the rights, values and privacy of the participants.

Once the protocol had been validated, we approached the dean's office to request the research, then sought the agreement of the chief medical officer of the Baco-Djicoroni AScom, and then the Baco-Djicoroni district chief was informed of the survey so that we could obtain his verbal authorisation to investigate.

Respect for medical ethics and deontology is an integral part of this study, which has endeavoured to respect the following aspects:

- information for verbal, individual, free and informed consent from participants, and a form has been drawn up for participants to this end,
- respect for people's opinions and decisions, with informed and appropriate information,
- guaranteed anonymity and confidentiality.

Chapter 6

RESULTS

6. Results

At the end of this study, a quantitative survey was carried out with 660 individuals in the six sectors of the Baco-Djicoroni neighbourhood (Sokoura, Dougoukoro, Hèrèmakono, Plateau, ACI and Golf), i.e. 110 individuals per sector, and a qualitative survey (focus group) with a group of 6 individuals in 3 sectors (Dougoukoro, Sokoura and ACI).

The results obtained are presented in two (2) phases depending on the type of study (qualitative and quantitative).

6.1.Socio-demographic characteristics

During this study, the questionnaire was administered to the 660 participants.

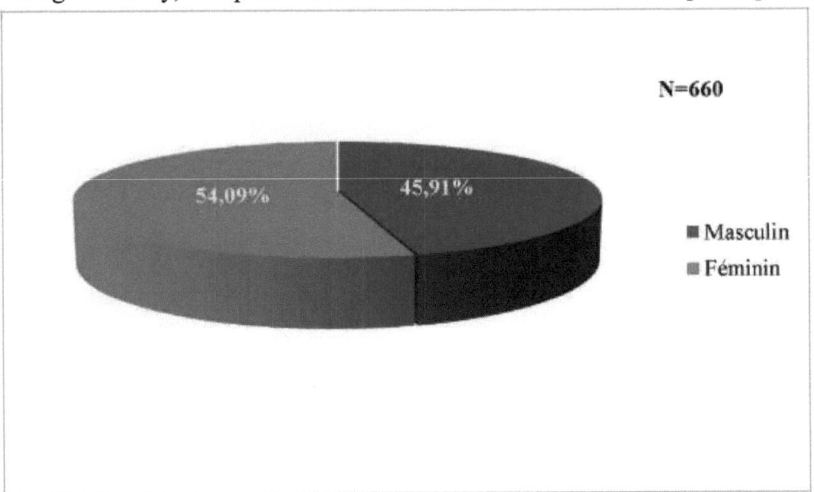

Figure 5: Distribution of respondents by gender

Analysis of the results showed a slight predominance of women (54.09%) (Figure 5).

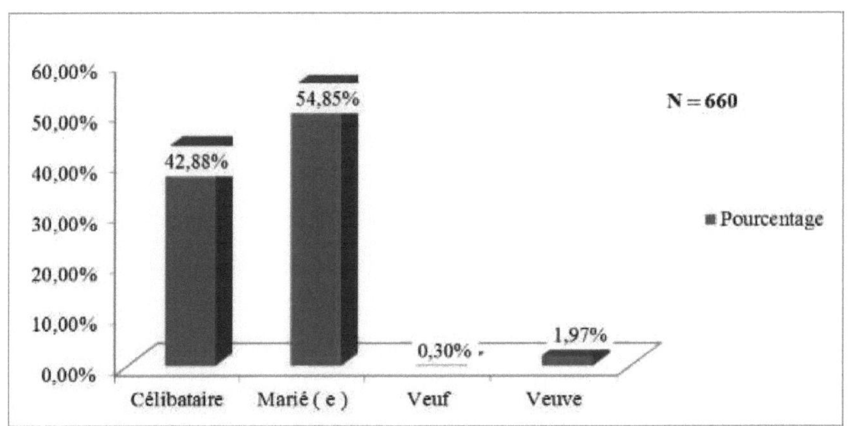

Figure 6: Distribution of respondents by marital status

In the study, married people were the most represented, at 54.85% (Figure 6).

Table VI: Distribution of respondents by profession

Profession	Workforce	Frequency (%)
Civil servant	**154**	**23,33**
Housekeeper	124	18,79
Student	116	17,58
Retailer	103	15,61
Worker	74	11,21
Student	55	8,33
Other	22	3,33
Retired civil servant	12	1,82
TOTAL	660	100

Civil servants were the most represented, with a total of 154, or 23.33% (Table VI).

Table VII: Distribution of respondents by religion

Religion	Workforce	Frequency (%)
Muslim woman	**631**	**95,61**
Christian	27	4,09
Traditional	2	0,30
TOTAL	660	100

Muslims were the most represented with 95.61% (Table VII).

Table VIII: Distribution of respondents by ethnic group

Ethnic group	Workforce	Frequency (%)

Bambara	**194**	**29,39**
Malinké	103	15,61
Peulh	97	14,70
Soninké	67	10,15
Dogon	35	5,30
Sonrhaï	34	5,15
Minianka	31	4,70
Senoufo	27	4,09
Bwa	18	2,73
Bozo	17	2,58
Khassonké	17	2,58
Not specified	11	1,67
Tamacheck	4	0,61
Mossi	3	0,45
Maure	2	0,30
TOTAL	660	100

The Bambara ethnic group was the most represented with 29.39%, followed by the Malinkés with 15.61% and the Peulhs with 14.70% (Table VIII).

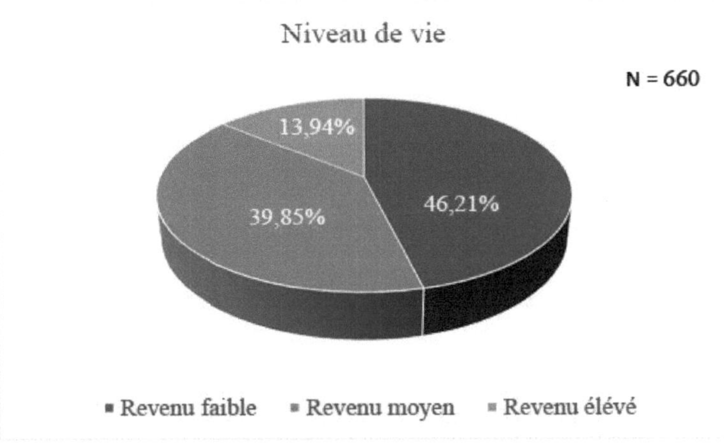

Figure 7: Distribution of respondents by standard of living

In the study, 305 respondents (46.21%) considered their standard of living to be low (Figure 7).

Table IX: Distribution of respondents by sector according to income

Standard of living	Low income		Average income		High income		TOTAL	
	n	%	n	%	n	%	n	%
Tray	**75**	**68,18**	31	28,18	4	3,64	110	100

Sokoura	**57**	**51,82**	43	39,09	10	9,09	110	100
Dougoukoro	**56**	**50,91**	46	41,82	8	7,27	110	100
Hèrèmakono	**53**	**48,18**	50	45,45	7	6,37	110	100
Golf	34	30,9	**49**	**44,55**	27	24,55	110	100
ACI	30	27,27	**44**	**40**	36	32,73	110	100

Average income was mentioned most by respondents in the Golf and ACI sectors (44.55% and 40% respectively), followed by low income in the Golf (30.90%) and high income in the ACI (32.73%), while low income was mentioned by more than half the respondents in the Plateau, Sokoura, Dougoukoro and Hèrèmakono sectors (68.18%, 51.82%, 50.91% and 48.18% respectively); Sokoura, Dougoukoro and Hèrèmakono (68.18%, 51.82%, 50.91% and 48.18% respectively) and a sizeable proportion reported having a medium income (28.18%, 39.09%, 41.82% and 45.45% respectively) (Table IX).

6.2.Knowledge about malaria

Tableau X: Distribution of respondents by sector according to their source of information on malaria

Knowledge of sources of information	Sokoura		Hèrèmakono		ACI		Golf		Dougoukoro		Tray	
	n	%	n	%	n	%	n	%	n	%	n	%
Media	**47**	**42,73**	**45**	**40,91**	**52**	**47,27**	**41**	**37,27**	**38**	**34,55**	**47**	**42,73**
Nursing staff	23	20,91	24	21,82	23	20,91	18	16,36	24	21,82	22	20
Internet	12	10,91	9	8,18	8	7,27	10	9,09	8	7,27	8	7,27
With the family	12	10,91	14	12,73	13	11,82	24	21,82	15	13,64	14	12,73
Personal experience	8	7,27	6	5,45	2	1,82	8	7,27	10	9,09	9	8,18
The school	8	7,27	12	19,91	12	10,91	9	8,18	15	13,64	10	9,09
TOTAL	110	100	110	100	110	100	110	100	110	100	110	100

*Media: Television, radio, newspapers, etc.

Respondents in all sectors received information about malaria from the media (TV, radio, newspapers, etc.).), i.e. 47.27% in ACI; 42.73% in Sokoura and Plateau; 40.91% in Hèrèmakono; 37.27% in Golf and 34.55% in Dougoukoro, followed by nursing staff in the Dougoukoro and Hèrèmakono sectors, i.e. 21.82%; Sokoura and ACI, i.e. 20.91 and Plateau, i.e. 20.00 and then followed by the family in the Golf sector, i.e. 21.82% (Table X).

Tableau XI: Distribution of respondents by sector according to knowledge of signs (all signs combined) of malaria by sector

Knowledge of signs	Positive responses (Total respondents)	Frequency (%)
ACI	70 (110)	63,63
Sokoura	66 (110)	60,00
Hèrèmakono	62 (110)	56,36
Dougoukoro	56 (110)	50,91
Golf	49 (110)	44,55
Tray	48 (110)	43,64

Respondents in all sectors were aware of the signs of malaria, but each sector had a specific frequency that differed from the others, with ACI 70 (110) or 63.63%, Sokoura 66 (110) or 60.00%, Hèrèmakono 62 (110) or 56.36%, Dougoukoro 56 (110) or 50.91%, Golf 49 (110) or 44.55% and Plateau 48 (110) or 43.64% respectively (Table XI).

Tableau XII: Distribution of respondents according to knowledge of specific signs of malaria

Knowledge of signs	Positive responses (total respondents)	Frequency (%)
Fever	394(660)	59,7
Headaches	392(660)	59,39
Vomiting	307(660)	46,52
Curvature	177(660)	26,82
Anorexia	155(660)	23,48
Asthenia	140(660)	21,21
Thrill	128(660)	19,39

In the study, fever was mentioned by 394/660 or 59.7% of respondents, while 392/660 or 59.39% of respondents mentioned headaches followed by vomiting with 307/660 or 46.52% as signs of malaria (Table XII).

Tableau XIII: Distribution of respondents according to knowledge of malaria transmission by sector

Transmission mode	ACI		Sokoura		Dougoukoro		Golf		Tray		Hèrèmakono	
	n	%	n	%	n	%	n	%	n	%	n	%
Mosquitoes	**85**	**77,27**	**74**	**67,27**	**74**	**67,27**	**73**	**66,36**	**67**	**60,91**	**70**	**63,64**
Mosquitoes and unsuitable food	10	9,09	12	10,91	13	11,82	19	17,27	17	15,45	13	11,82
Consumption	3	2,73	12	10,91	10	9,09	7	6,36	8	7,27	12	10,91

of unfit food												
Mosquitoes and dirty environments	5	4,55	6	5,45	9	8,18	6	5,45	7	6,36	6	5,45
Consumption of fresh milk and eggs	7	6,36	6	5,45	4	3,64	5	4,55	11	10	9	8,18
TOTAL	110	100	110	100	110	100	110	100	110	100	110	100

For the mode of transmission of malaria, mosquito bites were most frequently mentioned in all sectors: 67.27% in Sokoura, 67.27% in Dougoukoro, 63.64% in Hèrèmakono, 60.91% in Plateau, 66.36% in Golf and 77.27% in ACI; 66.36% in Golf and 77.27% in ACI, followed by mosquitoes and unsuitable food: 10.91% in Sokoura; 11.82% in Dougoukoro and Hèrèmakono; 15.45% in Plateau; 17.27% in Golf and 9.09% in ACI (Table XIII).

<u>Tableau XIV:</u> Distribution of respondents according to their knowledge of the malaria vector (female anopheles) by sector

Malaria vector	Female Anopheles		Does not know		Anopheles male		TOTAL	
	n	%	n	%	n	%	n	%
ACI	**72**	**65,45**	31	28,18	7	6,36	110	100
Sokoura	**63**	**57,27**	43	39,09	4	3,64	110	100
Hèrèmakono	**60**	**54,55**	47	42,73	3	2,73	110	100
Golf	**55**	**50**	52	47,27	3	2,73	110	100
Tray	50	45,45	**54**	**49,09**	6	5,45	110	100
Dougoukoro	46	41,82	**61**	**55,45**	3	2,73	110	100

Among the respondents, those from the ACI, Sokoura, Hèrèmakono and Golf sectors mentioned that the female anopheles causes malaria, with 65.45%, 57.27%, 54.55% and 50% respectively, followed by those who felt they did not know that the female anopheles is the vector of malaria, i.e. 28.18%; 39.09%; 42.73% and 47.27%, respondents in the Plateau and Dougoukoro sectors felt they did not know that the female anopheles was the vector of malaria with 49.09% and 55.45% respectively, followed by those who felt that the female anopheles caused malaria with 45.45% and 41.82% (Table XIV).

<u>Tableau XV:</u> Distribution of respondents by sector according to their knowledge of when the malaria mosquito bites

Stinging moment	The night	I do not know	Any time	TOTAL

	n	%	n	%	n	%	n	%
Sokoura	**59**	**53,64**	8	7,27	43	39,09	110	100
Dougoukoro	**58**	**52,73**	7	6,36	45	40,91	110	100
Tray	**58**	**52,73**	12	10,91	40	36,36	110	100
Golf	51	46,36	4	3,64	**55**	**50**	110	100
ACI	**55**	**50**	8	7,27	47	42,73	110	100
Hèrèmakono	**54**	**49,09**	10	9,09	46	41,82	110	100

Respondents in the Sokoura, Dougoukoro, Plateau, Hèrèmakono and ACI sectors mentioned that malaria mosquitoes bite at night (53.64%, 52.73%, 52.73%, 50% and 49.09% respectively), followed by mosquitoes biting at any time (39.09%, 40.91%, 36.36%, 41.82% and 42.73%); 40.91%; 36.36%; 41.82% and 42.73%, while 50.00% of respondents in the Golf sector said that malaria mosquito vectors bite at any time, followed by mosquito bites at night (46.36%) (Table XV).

Table XVI: Distribution of respondents according to knowledge of the habitat of the malaria vector mosquito

Mosquito habitat	ACI		Sokoura		Dougoukoro		Tray		Hèrèmakono		Golf	
	n	%	n	%	n	%	n	%	n	%	n	%
Stagnant water and rubbish	**34**	**30,91**	**34**	**30,91**	33	30	30	27,27	28	25,45	27	24,55
Stagnant water	24	21,82	22	20	**34**	**30,91**	**37**	**33,64**	**30**	**27,27**	**30**	**27,27**
Rubbish	23	20,91	30	27,27	27	24,55	26	23,64	**30**	**27,27**	**30**	**27,27**
Don't know	26	23,64	20	18,18	12	10,91	13	11,82	15	13,64	19	17,27
Stagnant water, rubbish, dark area	3	2,73	4	3,64	4	3,64	4	3,64	7	6,36	4	3,64
TOTAL	110	100	110	100	110	100	110	100	110	100	110	100

Respondents in the Plateau, Dougoukoro, Golf and Hèrèmakono sectors mentioned stagnant water as the habitat of the malaria mosquito vector, with 33.64%, 30.91%, 27.27% and 27.27% respectively, while respondents in the ACI and Sokoura sectors mentioned stagnant water and rubbish as the habitat of the malaria mosquito vector, with 30.91% each (Table XVI).

Table XVII: Distribution of respondents according to knowledge of malaria prevention measures

Preventive measures	**Workforce**	**Frequency (%)**

Mosquito net	**302**	**45,76**
Mosquito nets, repellents and a clean environment	124	18,79
Mosquito nets and repellents	82	12,42
A clean environment	63	9,55
Preventive chemotherapy and mosquito nets	55	8,33
Repellents	19	2,88
Medicines	15	2,27
TOTAL	660	100

Mosquito nets were the means of prevention most used by the respondents (45.76%) (Table XVII).

<u>Table XVIII</u>: Distribution of respondents according to knowledge of malaria prevention measures by sector

Preventive measures	Dougoukoro		Tray		Sokoura		Hèrèmakono		Golf		ACI	
	n	%	n	%	n	%	n	%	n	%	n	%
Mosquito net	**53**	**48,18**	**52**	**47,27**	**51**	**46,36**	**51**	**46,36**	**50**	**45,45**	**45**	**40,91**
Mosquito nets, repellents and a clean environment	18	16,36	19	17,27	29	26,36	25	22,73	13	11,82	20	18,18
Mosquito net and repellents	13	11,82	14	12,73	11	10	6	5,45	19	17,27	19	17,27
Chemoprevention and mosquito nets	7	6,36	8	7,27	7	6,36	8	7,27	11	10	14	12,73
A clean environment	16	14,55	14	12,73	7	6,36	12	10,91	8	7,27	6	5,45
Medicines	3	2,73	3	2,73	3	2,73	5	4,55	0	0	1	0,91
Repellents	0	0	0	0	2	1,82	3	2,73	9	8,18	5	4,55
TOTAL	110	100	110	100	110	100	110	100	110	100	110	100

The mosquito net was the most frequently mentioned means of prevention in each sector: 48.18% in Dougoukoro; 47.27% in Plateau; 46.36% in Sokoura and Hèrèmakono; 45.45% in Golf and 40.91% in ACI (Table XVIII).

6.3. <u>Attitudes towards malaria</u>

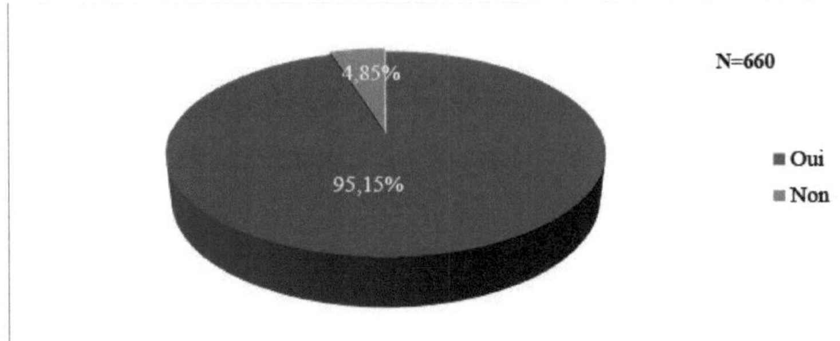

Figure 8: Distribution of respondents according to whether they consider malaria a serious threat to life

In the study, 628 respondents (95.15%) said that malaria was a serious threat to their lives (Figure 8).

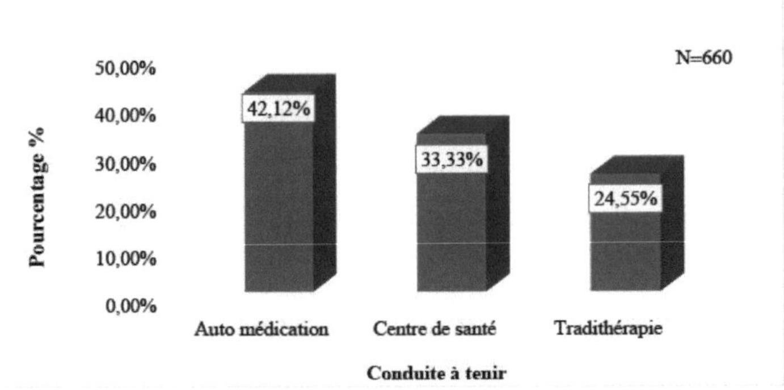

Figure 9: Distribution of respondents according to their attitudes to suspected malaria in terms of what to do In the study, 278 respondents (42.12%) resorted to self-medication in the event of malaria (Figure 9).

Table XIX: Distribution of respondents according to their attitudes to suspected malaria by sector in terms of action to be taken

What to do	Self-medication		Health centre		Traditherapy		TOTAL	
	n	%	n	%	n	%	n	%
Tray	**52**	**47,27**	33	30	25	22,73	110	100
ACI	**51**	**46,36**	41	37,27	18	16,36	110	100
Sokoura	**51**	**46,36**	34	30,91	25	22,73	110	100
Hèrèmakono	**48**	**43,64**	36	32,73	26	23,64	110	100
Dougoukoro	36	32,73	**39**	**35,45**	35	31,82	110	100
Golf	**40**	**36,36**	37	33,64	33	30	110	100

Respondents in the Plateau, Sokoura, ACI, Hèrèmakono and Golf sectors reported having more recourse to self-medication in cases of suspected malaria

(47.27%, 46.36%, 46.36%, 43.64% and 36.36% respectively), while respondents in the Dougoukoro sector reported having more recourse to the health centre in cases of malaria (35.45%), although 32.73% also reported having recourse to self-medication (Table XIX).

6.4. Malaria prevention practices

6.4.1. Possession of mosquito nets

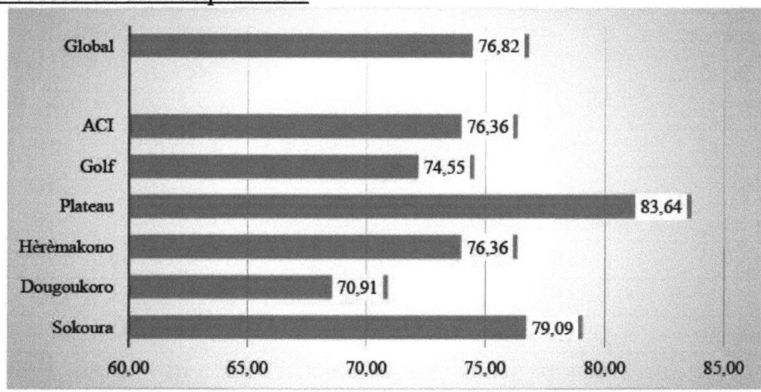

Figure 10: Distribution of respondents according to net ownership overall and by sector

Across all sectors, 76.82% confirmed that they had a mosquito net.

Respondents in all sectors mentioned having a mosquito net in their possession: 79.09% in Sokoura; 70.91% in Dougoukoro; 76.36% in Hèrèmakono; 83.64% in Plateau; 74.55% in Golf and 76.36% in ACI (Figure 10).

6.4.2. Use of mosquito nets

Tableau XX: Distribution of respondents according to frequency of use of mosquito nets by participants and their family members

Time categories	Workforce - Use by participants	Frequency (%)
Always	**309**	**46,82**
Often	168	25,45
Never	183	27,73
TOTAL	660	100
Time categories	**Workforce- Use by their families**	**Frequency (%)**
Always	**305**	**46,21**
Often	252	38,18

Never	103	15,61
TOTAL	660	100

Among the respondents, 72.27% said that they had used a mosquito net and 84.39% said that their family members used a mosquito net (Table XX).

Tableau XXI: **Distribution of respondents according to frequency of net use by sector**

Use of mosquito netting	Always		Often		Never		TOTAL	
	n	%	n	%	n	%	n	%
Tray	**60**	**54,55**	26	23,64	24	21,82	110	100
Sokoura	**56**	**50,91**	25	22,73	29	26,73	110	100
Golf	**54**	**49,09**	22	20	34	30,91	110	100
Dougoukoro	**50**	**45,45**	23	20,91	37	33,64	110	100
ACI	**45**	**40,91**	40	36,36	25	22,73	110	100
Hèrèmakono	**44**	**40**	32	29,09	34	30,91	110	100

Respondents in all sectors use a mosquito net: 78.19% in Plateau, 77.27% in ACI, 73.64% in Sokoura, 69.09% in Hèrèmakono and Golf and 66.36% in Dougoukoro (Table XXI).

Tableau XXII: **Distribution of respondents according to the use of mosquito nets by family members, by sector**

Use of mosquito nets by family members	Always		Often		Never		TOTAL	
	n	%	n	%	n	%	n	%
Tray	**70**	**63,64**	32	29,09	8	7,27	110	100
Sokoura	**54**	**49,09**	45	40,91	11	10	110	100
Golf	**51**	**46,36**	35	31,82	24	21,82	110	100
Dougoukoro	**51**	**46,36**	36	32,73	23	20,91	110	100
Hèrèmakono	43	39,09	**47**	**42,73**	20	18,18	110	100
ACI	36	32,73	**57**	**51,82**	17	15,45	110	100

Among the respondents, 92.73% mentioned that their family members use mosquito nets in the Plateau sector; 90.00% in Sokoura; 84.55% in ACI; 81.82% in Hèrèmakono; 79.09% in Dougoukoro; and 78.18% in Golf (Table XXII).

6.4.3. Checking the condition of mosquito nets

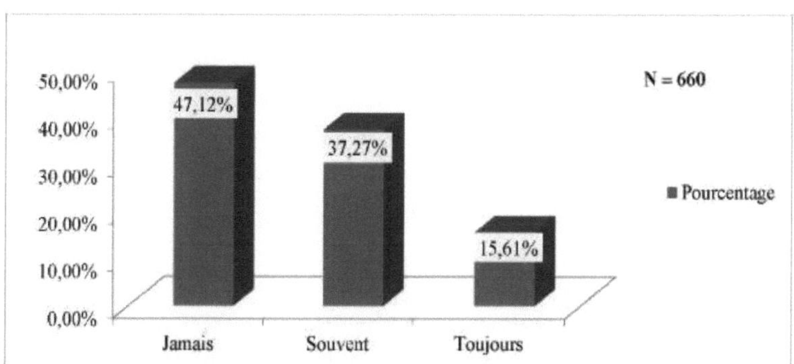

Figure 11: Distribution of respondents by verification of net condition

In the study, 311 respondents (47.12%) said they never checked the condition of their nets (Figure 11).

Table XXIII: Distribution of respondents by checking the condition of nets by sector

Checking the condition of mosquito nets	Never		Often		Always		TOTAL	
	n	%	n	%	n	%	n	%
Tray	**57**	**51,82**	43	39,09	10	9,09	110	100
Golf	**57**	**51,82**	30	27,27	23	20,91	110	100
Dougoukoro	**52**	**47,27**	44	40	14	12,73	110	100
Hèrèmakono	**49**	**44,55**	44	40	17	15,45	110	100
ACI	**49**	**44,55**	46	41,82	15	13,64	110	100
Sokoura	**47**	**42,73**	39	35,45	24	21,82	110	100

Respondents in all sectors said they never checked the condition of their nets: 51.82% in Plateau and Golf; 47.27% in Dougoukoro; 44.55% in Hèrèmakono and ACI; and 42.73% in Sokoura (Table XXIII).

6.5 Focus group

In this study, three (3) focus group interviews were carried out, one for each of 3 sectors, namely Dougoukoro, Sokoura and the ACI, distributed as follows: Six (6) participants living in the ACI (including a 46-year-old customs officer, a 62-year-old pensioner, a 65-year-old engineer, two housewives aged 49 and 40 and a 21-year-old student).

Six (6) participants living in Sokoura (including one 72-year-old, two housewives aged 41 and 25, two shopkeepers aged 41 and 49 and one small shopkeeper aged 23).

Six (6) participants living in Dougoukoro (including two students aged 25 and 31; two workers aged 36 and 29; a painter aged 27 and an accountant aged 33).

6.5.1. Knowledge of malaria

Recognising the signs of malaria

Opinions about malaria varied. The majority of respondents knew the signs of malaria. Many recognised malaria through signs such as fever, headaches and vomiting (Box 1). This result confirms the high frequency of knowledge of the signs of malaria in the quantitative analysis.

Box 1

"I recognise malaria in a person when they have a fever, repeated headaches and aches and pains" [Housewife, 41, Sokoura]. "I recognise malaria through vomiting and fever" [Retired 62-year-old, ACI].

"I recognise malaria in a person when they have a fever, are shivering and have aches and pains" [Accountant, 33, Dougoukoro].

Other terms for malaria

Most people call malaria "sumaya", while others call it "sayi" or "kônô" in the vernacular language of Bamanankan (Box 2).

Box 2

"Malaria is called 'sumaya'" [31-year-old student, Dougoukoro].

"Malaria is called 'sayi' or 'sayi djaima'" [72-year-old, Sokoura].

"Malaria is called 'sumaya', others say 'kônô' but also 'djokadjo'" [Customs officer, 46, ACI].

Difference between presentations of malaria in children and adults

The majority thought that children were the most vulnerable to malaria because they were unable to say what was wrong with them. Even before their parents realise they are ill, they find that they have been badly affected, whereas adults know as soon as they are ill and take precautions to ensure better care. This is confirmed by the quotes from the various respondents reported below (Box 3).

Box 3

"The only difference is that a child can't say that I'm ill, whereas an adult can say that my body is like this; it heats up; I'm too tired or I've got this. [Student, 25, Dougoukoro].

"Children are feverish in the morning and evening, they doze off a lot and have stomach aches, but adults have frequent headaches and dizziness and salivate a lot" [49-year-old shopkeeper, Sokoura].

"Yes, there's a difference, children can't say they're ill, but adults know when they're ill and that it's malaria" [Housewife, 49, ACI].

Factors favouring malaria

Participants thought that mosquito bites were the most cited cause of malaria, but others thought that in addition to mosquito bites, eating certain foods (containing oil, eggs, milk, etc.) could cause malaria (Box 4).

Box 4
"Malaria is caused by the bite of mosquitoes (female Anopheles)" [21-year-old student, ACI].
"I think it's mosquitoes that transmit malaria and eating food containing oil" [Tradeswoman, 41, Sokoura].
"Malaria is transmitted through food" [36-year-old worker, Dougoukoro].

Mosquitoes that transmit malaria

Most of the respondents thought that all mosquitoes could transmit malaria, while others thought that only the female Anopheles could transmit malaria (Box 5).

Box 5
"No, it's the female anopheles that transmits malaria" [Painter, 27, Dougoukoro].
"Yes, all mosquitoes can transmit malaria" [small business, 23, Sokoura].
"No, only the female anopheles can cause malaria" [Housewife, 40, ACI].

Protection against malaria

All the respondents were aware of ways of preventing malaria (Box 6). The shopkeepers and housewives had a general knowledge of sleeping under an insecticide-treated mosquito net and cleaning the environment. Students, private-sector employees and civil servants knew more, listing sleeping under a mosquito net, using repellents, environmental sanitation and chemoprevention.

Box 6
"You have to sleep under an impregnated mosquito net" [49-year-old housewife, ACI].
"I use mosquito nets and repellents" [Painter, 27, Dougoukoro].
"Let's get everyone together to sweep up, clean up the environment and prevent the water from stagnating. Stagnant water is what breeds mosquitoes, and it's mosquitoes that transmit malaria. Let's work together to clean up the environment and avoid stagnant water, then attach mosquito nets" [Housewife, 41, Sokoura].

6.5.2. <u>Attitudes in the event of malaria</u>

Attitudes towards cases of suspected malaria

Attitudes varied (Box 7), with most respondents adopting an attitude of self-medication followed by consultation with a doctor. Some used medicinal plants.

Box 7
"I start with paracetamol, and if it doesn't work, I go to a health centre with traditional medicines" [Housewife, 41, Sokoura].
"I take tablets if they don't help, I go to a health centre" [Student, 21, ACI].
"I start with treatment, whether it's pharmaceutical or traditional medicines to combat malaria" [Worker, 36, Dougoukoro].

Choosing one person to sleep under a mosquito net if there was only one

Most respondents said that sleeping under mosquito nets was a priority for children (Box 8).

Box 8

"I make the children sleep" [Worker, 29, Dougoukoro].
"I make children and pregnant women sleep" [customs officer, 46, ACI].
"We all go inside to sleep" [25-year-old housewife, Sokoura].

6.5.3. Practices in the event of malaria

What to do if you suspect malaria

Most of the respondents were self-medicating (Box 9). After having tried all kinds of treatment without success, they went to a health centre, while others continued to use traditional medicines as well as being treated in a health centre. Once at the health centre, many continued the treatment prescribed by the doctors until they were cured, while sleeping under a mosquito net.

Box 9

"I buy anti-malaria drugs in a pharmacy, particularly coartem, and I fill my stomach with them for 3 days" [Student, 25, Dougoukoro].

"I prepare traditional medicines; even if I give him serum in a health centre, I continue to give him medicinal plants to drink and at home the children always sleep under mosquito nets" [Tradeswoman, 49, Sokoura].

"Do first aid in a health centre and get the patient to eat by filling his stomach, but avoid certain foods containing oil and avoid drinking milk" [Engineer, 65, ACI].

The need to sleep under an insecticide-treated mosquito net

Opinions on the need to sleep under a mosquito net were mixed (Box 10). Most participants said that it was very important to sleep under a mosquito net and that it was a means of preventing malaria. Other participants, however, said that it was more necessary to live in a clean environment; in their opinion, as long as the environment was unhealthy, it would be difficult to eradicate malaria.

Box 10

"No, because it only protects us when we go to sleep, whereas we spend more time outdoors" [Retired 62, ACI].

"Yes, it's very important, it protects us and our children against malaria" [shopkeeper, 23, Sokoura].

"Yes, it's very important, it protects you against malaria" [Accountant, 33, Dougoukoro].

Chapter 7

COMMENTS AND DISCUSSION

7. Comments and discussion

7.1. Socio-demographic data

- **Gender**

In this study, 54.09% of participants were female. This female predominance was also reported by TAGNE L in 2021, who found that in Koulouba, 78Sogonafing and Point G the female sex was the most represented at 50.86% [47], and contrary to that of TRAORE A in 2020, who found that in Kalifabougou the male sex was the most represented at 56.30% [31]. This difference could be explained by the frequency of women in households at the time of the study data collection.

- **Marital status and occupation**

During the study, the majority of respondents (54.85%) were married. This result is lower than that found by KEITA A in a study also conducted in Baco-Djicoroni in 2012, where 85.50% of respondents were married [48].

Civil servants dominated the study with 23.33%. This result is different from that found in 2013 by SAMAKE OS in commune 5 of the Bamako district where 56.70% were housewives [49].

This difference could be explained by the fact that data collection for the study was carried out even at weekends, and many civil servants were present at home.

7.2. Knowledge about malaria

- **Sources of information**

One of the main sources of information about malaria for the population was the media (TV, radio, newspapers, etc.) with 40.59%. This result was lower than that of GOITA A in the Baguineda health area in 2010 with 46.00% [50]; and is also different from that of the study carried out by KEITA A in the district of Baco-Djicoroni in 2012 with 53.50% [48]. This difference in figures is due to the fact that the media such as television, radio, etc. (which are accessible to many people) do not sufficiently disseminate information on malaria and are no longer followed as they used to be. (which are accessible to many people) do not sufficiently disseminate information about malaria and are no longer followed as they used to be.

- **Signs of malaria**

Fever was the sign of malaria most evoked by participants with 59.70%, followed by headaches with 59.39% and vomiting 46.52%. DIALLO R found in his study carried out in Niamakoro in 2018 for the signs of malaria, that headaches were the sign most evoked by participants with 93.40%, followed by fever with 90.20% and vomiting with 88.00% [12].

In a study carried out in Koulouba, Sogonafing and Point G by TAGNE L in 2021, fever was the sign most frequently mentioned by participants (94.54%), followed by headaches (80.46%) and general fatigue (70.97%) [47].

- **Knowledge of the mode of transmission**

In the study, mosquito bites were mentioned by 67.12% of participants, followed by mosquito bites and food consumption (12.73%).

GOITA MK found in Ouéléssébougou in 2012 that mosquito bites were cited by 54.40% of participants, followed by the consumption of fatty foods cited by 38.20% [11]. TAGNE L, found in Koulouba, Sogonafing and Point g in 2021 that mosquito bites were cited by 99.43% and the consumption of unfit food was cited by 54.31% [47]. COULIBALY IH found in 2012 in the rural commune of Bancoumana (commune located in the health district of Kati) that mosquito bites were cited by only 12.20% and 66.90% cited mosquito bites and fatty foods as the cause of malaria [51]. SAMAKE OS found in commune 5 of the Bamako district in 2013 that mosquito bites were cited by 31% and 22.5% cited mosquito bites and fatty foods [49].

- **Knowledge of prevention measures**

In the present study, 45.68% of participants mentioned mosquito nets as the most commonly used means of preventing malaria, followed by the use of mosquito nets, repellents and a clean environment with 18.82%. TAGNE L, found in his study in Koulouba, Sogonafing and Point G in 2021 that the mosquito net was the most commonly used means of prevention with 85.55%, followed by the use of mosquito repellent spirals with 69.65% and cleaning the surroundings of the house with 67.34%, then only 13.22% did not have a mosquito net [47]. GOITA MK found in his study in Ouéléssébougou in 2012 that 80.75% of subjects had slept under a mosquito net the night before the survey [11].

This difference can be explained by the fact that the participants in this study would use other means of protection against malaria apart from the mosquito net, and also that not all of them would own a mosquito net.

7.3. Attitudes towards malaria

- **Malaria as a serious threat to life**

The results of the survey showed that 95.15% of those questioned considered malaria to be a serious threat to life. They described it as a serious and fatal disease. In DIALLO R's study in the peri-urban district of Niamakoro (Bamako, Mali) in 2018, 97.8% of participants had perceived malaria as a serious and fatal disease [12].

- **What to do**

In the study, 42.12% of participants resorted first to self-medication if they suspected malaria, followed by 33.33% who went to the health centre and 24.55% who resorted to traditional therapy. In her 2019 study in Ségou, FANE B found that 38.20% of the mothers surveyed cited traditional self-medication as their first recourse in the event of malaria. This could be explained by the strong dominance of their cultural beliefs [52]. DIALLO R found in his 2018 study that 91.80% of participants had recourse to the nearest health centre in the event of malaria, followed by 78.50% for paracetamol and 49.90% for a modern antimalarial [12]. SAGARA A, in his study in Fana in 2018, found that 90.20% of the mothers surveyed used the health centre in the event of malaria and 54.00% gave better treatment as the reason [53].

In their 2000 study in Benin, Kiniffo et al found that 80.20% of respondents used the health centre in the event of severe malaria; 1.5% used traditional healers and 17.70% recommended prayers or continuing treatment at home [54]. This difference in figures is due to the fact that the study focused on adults, the majority of whom prefer to self-medicate as a first resort if they suspect malaria, unlike children (0-5 years) who are more vulnerable to malaria and whose mothers prefer to go directly to the health centre for better treatment and recovery.

7.4.Practical for prevention

- Use of mosquito netting

Almost all the participants were unanimous about the effectiveness, importance and place of insecticide-treated mosquito nets, indoor residual spraying, the use of repellents and chemoprevention in malaria prevention. In the study, 72.27% of participants said they had used mosquito nets.

TRAORE MK found in 2013in Samè in commune III of the district of Bamako in his sample that 80.20% of participants used mosquito nets, of which 254 or 98.10% used insecticide-treated nets [55]. SANGARE M during his study in Samè in commune III of the district of Bamako found in 2013 that 71.1% of participants used insecticide-treated nets and 14.5% of participants used simple mosquito nets [56].

7.5.Limits of the study

A prospective cross-sectional study was carried out on the knowledge, attitudes and practices of the population of the Baco-Djicoroni health area regarding malaria prevention. However, there are some limitations to the survey. There was a possibility of information bias because the respondents were not directly observed on their practices, but according to their declarations. During the survey period, the first difficulty encountered was the refusal of some residents to participate because they could not obtain mosquito nets or money before the interview. Also, the number of participants taken in each sector should be proportional to the number of inhabitants in each sector, whereas this study took an equal value for all sectors.

Chapter 8

CONCLUSION AND RECOMMENDATIONS

8. Conclusion and recommendations

Conclusion

The study population in Baco-Djicoroni perceived malaria as a serious and fatal disease. The most frequent sign was fever; the standard of living, with low and average incomes, was most frequently mentioned by the population in relation to their daily and monthly expenses. In practice, the study population said they protected themselves from malaria by using mosquito nets. Self-medication was the first recourse to care among the study population. In the event of failure, the population turned to the health centres.

Recommendations

Ministry of Health and Social Development :

- Diversify communication channels in the fight against malaria, in particular by adding social networks;
- Increase the dissemination of information on malaria prevention methods via radio, television and newspapers.

The National Malaria Control Programme (PNLP):

- Strengthen public awareness campaigns to promote the use of impregnated mosquito nets;
- CCC on the benefits of using insecticide-treated mosquito nets ;
- Making mosquito nets more accessible to local people.

To healthcare providers :

- Continue to raise public awareness of malaria prevention methods and early recourse to health services;
- Set up a door-to-door awareness and information team on malaria transmission and prevention methods.

To the public:

- Avoid self-medication if malaria is suspected;
- Go to the health centre as soon as fever or other signs of malaria appear;

❖ Sanitise living areas, sleep under a mosquito net;

❖ Adhere to the preventive measures recommended by the national malaria control programme.

REFERENCES

[1] World Health Organization, "Global Technical Strategy for Malaria 2016-2030", 2015. https://www.who.int/fr/publications-detail/9789241564991 (consulted on 5 January 2023).

[2] BOURGEOIS Evelyne, "Malaria (ANOFEL) Association Française des Enseignants de Parasitologie et Mycologie 2014", *Article*, 2014. https://fr.readkong.com/page/paludisme-association-francaise-des- enseignants-de-6695706 (accessed 19 January 2023).

[3] WHO, "Report of the Ministerial Conference on Malaria, Amsterdam, 26-27 October 1992", *Report*, October 1992. https://apps.who.int/iris/handle/10665/58663 (consulted on 11 January 2023).

[4] TRAORE Yaya Toumani, "Inventaire des répulsifs anti moustiques dans le district de Bamako, MALI", *Thèse Pharmacie*, 2012. https://www.bibliosante.ml/handle/123456789/1447?show=full (accessed 23 January 2023).

[5] TRAORE. D. COULIBALY. D. DOUMBO. O. KYALO. D. MAINA. J. K. MACHARIA. P. M. OKIRO. E. A. SNOW. R. W. THURANIIRA. P. N. GIORGI. E. D. N. H. L. L. R. L. C. KONATE.M, "Profil de l'épidémiologie et de la lutte contre le paludisme au MALI", *Report*, 2018.

[6] WHO, "Malaria", *Report*, 2021. https://www.who.int/fr/news- room/fact-sheets/detail/malaria (accessed 16 January 2023).

[7] WHO, "The Impact of Our Projects: Accelerating Access to Seasonal Malaria Chemoprevention", *Report*, 2012.

[8] WHO (World Health Organization), "World Malaria Report 2022", *Report*, 2022. https://www.who.int/publications/i/item/9789240064898 (consulted on 10 July 2023).

[9] Institut National de la Statistique (INSTAT), "Mali - Enquête Démographique et de Santé 2018", *report*, 2019. https://microdata.worldbank.org/index.php/catalog/3526 (consulted on 11 April 2023).

[10] GOUTILLE Fabienne, "Connaissances, attitudes et pratiques dans l'éducation au risque : mettre en oeuvre les études CAP : guide à l'intention des chefs de projet pour les études CAP", *Article*, October 2009. https://catalogue.bnf.fr/ark:/12148/cb42265258d (accessed 16 January 2023).

[11] GOITA Moussa K, " Connaissance, attitudes et pratique des populations face au paludisme à " Ouélésséobougou " de Novembre 2009 à Août 2011 ",

Thèse Médecine, 2012.
https://www.bibliosante.ml/handle/123456789/1415?show=full (consulted on 11 January 2023).
[12] DIALLO Rapha, "Connaissances, attitudes et pratiques de la population face au paludisme dans un quartier péri urbain de Bamako : Niamakoro", *Thèse Médecine*, 2018. https://bibliosante.ml/handle/123456789/2037 (accessed 11 January 2023).
[13] World Health Organization, "World malaria report 2021", *Report*, 2021. https://www.who.int/teams/global-malaria- programme/reports/world-malaria-report-2021 (consulted on 11 January 2023).
[14] GUINDO Banou, "Etude de la dispensation des médicaments dans les officines de Bamako", *Thèse Pharmacie*, 2021.
https://bibliosante.ml/handle/123456789/4710 (consulted on 11 January 2023).
[15] Le Robert, "Definition - Knowledge, Le petit Robert de la langue française 2023", *Book*, 20 September 2022.
https://dictionnaire.lerobert.com/definition/connaissance (consulted on 31 July 2023).
[16] Le Robert, "Definition - Attitude, Le petit Robert de la langue française 2023", *Online dictionary*, 20 September 2022.
https://dictionnaire.lerobert.com/definition/attitude (consulted on 31 July 2023).
[17] Le Robert, "Definition - Pratique, Le petit Robert de la langue française 2023", *online dictionary*, 20 September 2022.
https://dictionnaire.lerobert.com/definition/pratique (consulted on 31 July 2023).
[18] Présidence de la république du MALI, "Mali - Loi n° 02-049/ du 22 juillet 2002 portant loi d'orientation sur la santé", *Article*, April 2008.
https://www.ilo.org/dyn/natlex/natlex4.detail?p_lang=fr&p_isn=96993
(accessed 16 January 2023).
[19] B. G. T. D. BOURDILLON François, "Santé / Prévention - Définition du concept de " Prévention en Santé Publique " | AP-HM", *Edition Médecine-Sciences Flammarion.* http://fr.ap-hm.fr/sante- prevention/definition-concept (accessed 16 January 2023).
[20] SAMASSA Famory, "Etude de la saisonnalité du paludisme à Plasmodium falciparum en milieu urbain de Bamako", *Thèse Médecine*, 2010.
[21] PNLP, "Plan Stratégique de Lutte Contre le Paludisme 2013-2017", August 2013.
[22] COULIBALY Bacoura Issaka, "Connaissance attitude et pratique face au paludisme de la population du village de Nanguilabougou et aux environnants, commune rurale de à Bancoumana (Mali", *Thèse Médecine*, 2012. https://www.bibliosante.ml/handle/123456789/1386 (accessed 11 January

2023).
[23] O.-P. E. C. V Pages F, "Malaria vectors: biology, diversity, control and individual protection - EM consults", *Medicine and Infectious Diseases*, 2007. https://www.em-consulte.com/article/60272/vecteurs- du-paludisme-biologie-diversite-controle- (consulted on 11 January 2023).
[24] Tropical medicine, "Major endemics News 2016 Professor Pierre Aubry, Doctor Bernard-Alex Gaüzère. Updated on 18/03/ PDF Free Download", 2021. https://docplayer.fr/23946022-Grandes-endemies- actualites-2016-professeur-pierre-aubry-docteur-bernard-alex-gauzere- mise-a-jour-le-18-03-2016.html (consulted on 11 January 2023).
[25] BEAVOGUI Abdoul Habib, "Role of apoptosis in the transmission of Plasmodium falciparum. Agricultural Sciences. Université Claude Bernard-Lyon I, 2010. French", *Thesis*, 2010. https://theses.hal.science/tel- 00825158 (accessed 11 January 2023).
[26] Sciensano, "AVIQ (Agency for a Quality Life): Malaria", *Article*, 2016.
[27] THOMAS Hélène, "Malaria news. Ce que doit savoir le pharmacien d'officine - Archive ouverte HAL", *Article*, March 2018. https://hal.univ-lorraine.fr/hal-01733720/ (accessed 19 January 2023).
[28] L. Ben Daoud, "Maludisme à plasmodium ovale: Expérience du service de médecine interne de l'Hôpital Militaire Avicenne de Marrakech", *Thesis*, 2018.
[29] M. Cissoko *et al*, "Stratification at the health district level for targeting malaria control interventions in Mali", *Scientific Reports 2022 12:1*, vol. 12, n° 1, p. 1-17, May 2022, doi: 10.1038/s41598-022-11974-3.
[30] CISSOKO Mady, "Etude de l'épidémiologie du paludisme en fonction des facteurs météorologiques et sociétaux au Mali", *Thesis*, 2022. https://www.theses.fr/2022AIXM0245 (accessed 11 April 2023).
[31] TRAORE Abdoulaye, "Etude épidémiologique du paludisme en 2019 dans une cohorte de volontaires à Kalifabougou", *Thèse Médecine*, 2020. https://www.bibliosante.ml/handle/123456789/4118?show=full (accessed 11 January 2023).
[32] Dr MENTA Djenebou TRAORE, "Cours en médecine sur le paludisme", *Med Interne*.
[33] PNLP, "DIRECTIVES NATIONALES POUR LA PRISE EN CHARGE DES CASES DE PALUDISME AU MALI", Mali, June 2016.
[34] TANGARA Abdoulaye, "Prescription et disponibilité des antipaludiques dans les Cscom de la commune urbaine de Kati", *Thèse Pharmacie*, 2006.
[35] SISSOKO Fadigui, "Attitude et pratique de personnel de santé devant les cas présumés de paludisme dans le CsCom de Torokorobougou et Quartier Mali

à Bamako", *Thèse Médecine*, 2014.
https://www.bibliosante.ml/handle/123456789/624 (consulted on 11 January 2023).
[36] WHO, "Implementation of malaria in pregnancy programmes in the context of World Health Organization (WHO) recommendations for antenatal care to make pregnancy a positive experience", *Report*, January 2018. https://apps.who.int/iris/handle/10665/259955 (accessed 11 January 2023).
[37] WHO Global Malaria Programme, "WHO policy recommendation: seasonal malaria chemoprevention to control Plasmodium falciparum malaria in areas of high seasonal transmission in the Sahel sub-region of Africa", *Report*, March 2012.
https://apps.who.int/iris/handle/10665/337982?show=full (consulted on 11 January 2023).
[38] METAIS. M. ,TRAORE. I. CHARPENTIER.P, " Diagnostic architectural, urbain et environnemental du [sous]quartier Fitribougou de Baco-Djicoroni à Bamako - MALI - PDF Téléchargement Gratuit ", *Article*, 2009. https://docplayer.fr/37227403-Diagnostic-architectural-urbain-et-environnemental-du-sous-quartier-fitribougou-de-baco-djicoroni-a- bamako-mali.html (accessed 11 January 2023).
[39] SurveyMonkey Audience, "Calculating the number of participants required | SurveyMonkey Help", *Article*.
https://help.surveymonkey.com/fr/surveymonkey/solutions/calculating-respondents/ (accessed 16 January 2023).
[40] Le Robert, "Definition - Standard of living, Le petit Robert de la langue française 2023", *Online dictionary*, 20 September 2022.
https://dictionnaire.lerobert.com/definition/niveau (consulted on 31 July 2023).
[41] J.-M. Hourriez and L. Olier, "Niveau de vie et taille du ménage : estimations d'une échelle d'équivalence", *Economie et Statistique*, vol. 308, n° 1, pp. 65-94, 1998, doi: 10.3406/ESTAT.1998.2591.
[42] Le Robert, "Definition - Revenu, Le petit Robert de la langue française 2023", *online dictionary*, 20 September 2022.
https://dictionnaire.lerobert.com/definition/revenu (consulted on 31 July 2023).
[43] Mladen Adamovic, "Salaire moyen au Mali", *numbeo*, April 2009. https://www.journaldunet.com/business/salaire/mali/pays-mli (accessed 23 February 2023).
[44] Government Activity Thesaurus, "Definition: Low Income Family", *TAG online*, 2000.
https://www.thesaurus.gouv.qc.ca/tag/terme.do?id=5429 (accessed 23 February 2023).

[45] Institut de la Statistique du Québec, "Revenu - Définitions et informations utiles". https://statistique.quebec.ca/fr/produit/publication/cdmi-revenu (consulted on 7 March 2023).
[46] Statistics Canada, "Appendix 3.1 Derived Statistics - Dictionary of the National Household Survey (NHS)," *Article*, 2011. https://www12.statcan.gc.ca/nhs-enm/2011/ref/dict/a3-1-fra.cfm (consulted on February 28, 2023).
[47] MEKOWA TAGNE Laurence Larissa, "Paludisme: connaissances, pratiques de prévention et itinéraires thérapeutiques à Koulouba, Sogonafing et Point G (Bamako, Mali)", *Thèse Médecine*, 2021. https://www.bibliosante.ml/handle/123456789/4599 (accessed 11 January 2023).
[48] KEITA Abdoulaye, "Prise en charge du paludisme présumé simple chez les enfants de 0-59 mois au centre de santé de Baco Djicoroni", *Thesis Medicine*, September 2012.
https://www.bibliosante.ml/handle/123456789/1419?show=full (consulted on 11 January 2023).
[49] SAMAKE Ousmane Sekou, "Etude des connaissances, attitudes, et pratiques des mères d'enfants de 0 à 59 mois sur le paludisme en commune V du district de Bamako", *Thèse Médecine*, 2013.
https://www.bibliosante.ml/handle/123456789/1784 (consulted on 11 January 2023).
[50] GOITA Aïssata, "Knowledge, attitudes and practices of populations in relation to malaria in the Baguineda health area", 2010.
[51] COULIBALY Issa Harouna, "Etude sur les connaissances, attitudes et pratiques des mères d'enfants de 0 à 59 mois sur le paludisme dans la commune rurale de Bancoumana", *Thesis Medicine*, 2012.
https://www.bibliosante.ml/handle/123456789/1406 (consulted on 11 January 2023).
[52] FANE Bakary, "Evaluation de la prise en charge du paludisme chez les enfants de 0 à 59 mois admis dans le centre de santé communautaire de Farako", *Thèse Médecine*, 2019.
https://www.bibliosante.ml/handle/123456789/4285 (consulted on 11 January 2023).
[53] SAGARA Abdramane, "Etude des connaissances, attitudes, et pratiques des mères d'enfants de 0 à 59 mois sur le paludisme dans la commune urbaine de Fana", *Thesis Medicine*, 2018.
https://www.bibliosante.ml/handle/123456789/1943?show=full (consulted on 11 January 2023).

[54] I. R. KINIFFO, L. AGBO-OLA, S. ISSIFOU, and A. MASSOUGBODJI, " Les mères des enfants de moins de cinq ans et le paludisme dans la vallée de Dangbo au sud-est du Benin ", *Med Afr Noire*, vol. 47, n° 1, p. 27-33, 2000.

[55] TRAORE Mahamadou Kassa, "Utilisation des moustiquaires imprégnées d'insecticide et la survenue du paludisme au sein des ménages de Samé en commune III du district de Bamako", *Thèse Médecine*, 2013. https://www.bibliosante.ml/handle/123456789/684 (consulted on 11 January 2023).

[56] SANGARE Marguérite, "Stratégies de lutte contre le paludisme: utilisation des moustiquaires imprégnées d'insectes au sein des ménages de Samé en commune III du district de Bamako", 2013.

10. Appendices

Material Safety Data Sheet

Last name: TRAORE **First name:** RAMATA YAKARE

Email: **ramatayakaretraore@!gmail.com** **Telephone:** (+223) 73456730

Title of thesis: Knowledge, attitudes and practices of the population of the Baco-Djicoroni health area regarding malaria prevention.

Academic year : 2021-2022 **City of defence :** Bamako

Country of origin: MALI **Place of deposit:** FMOS Library

Areas of interest: Public health, social sciences and prevention ethics.

Summary

This was a prospective cross-sectional study of the knowledge, attitudes and preventive practices of people in the Baco-Djicoroni health area.

The cross-sectional study, involving 660 adults aged 18 and over, was carried out from June 2021 to November 2021. Its aim was to assess the knowledge, attitudes and practices of people in the Baco-Djicoroni health area regarding malaria prevention.

The study covered residents of Sokoura, Hèrèmakono, Dougoukoro, Plateau, Golf and ACI. A questionnaire was administered to 110 people per sector for at least 6 months. We selected families at random and interviewed each person individually and separately to avoid any influence from one family to another. As for the focus group interview guide, with the permission of the participants, the interviews were recorded using a dictaphone.

We interviewed 357 women (54.09%) and 303 men (45.91%).

The standard of living with a low income was most frequently mentioned in four sectors: Plateau (68.18%), Sokoura (51.82%), Dougoukoro (50.91%) and Hèrèmakono (48.18%): Golf (44.55%) and ACI (40.00%).

Fever (hot body) with 59.70% was the most frequent sign, followed by headaches with 59.39% and vomiting with 46.52%. Mosquito bites were the most frequently mentioned sign (67.12% of participants), followed by mosquito bites and the consumption of unfit food (12.73%). Most participants had a mosquito net (76.82%).

The first place to seek care was self-medication (42.12%), followed by a visit to a health centre (33.33%).

The mosquito net was the most commonly used method, accounting for 45.76%.

The population of Baco-Djicoroni perceived malaria as a serious and fatal disease and attributed most of the illness to mosquito bites. As a result, most people used insecticide-treated mosquito nets to prevent it.

Key words: **Malaria, knowledge, attitude, practice, health area, prevention.**

Signaletic file

Name: TRAORE **First name**: RAMATA YAKARE

Email address: ramatayakaretraore@gmail.com **Phone number**: (+223)73456730

Title of thesis: knowledge, attitudes and practices of the populations of the Baco-Djicoroni health area on the prevention of malaria

Academic year: 2021-2022 **City of defense**: Bamako

Country of origin: Mali **Place of deposit**: FMOS library

Sectors of interest: public health, social sciences and prevention ethics.

Abstract

This was a prospective cross-sectional study on the knowledge, attitudes and prevention practices of populations in the Baco-Djicoroni health area.

The cross-sectional study, involving 660 adults aged 18years and over, was carried out from June 2021 to November 2021, that is a period of 6 months. Its objective was to assess the knowledge, attitudes and practices of the populations of the Baco-Djicoroni health area on the prevention of malaria.

The study concerned inhabitants residing either in Sokoura, Hèrèmakono, Dougoukoro, Plateau, Golf or ACI. A questionnaire was administered to 110 people per sector for at least 6 months. We selected families at random where all people were interviewed individually and separately to avoid influencing each other. Regarding the focus group interview guide, with the permission of the participants, the interviews were recorded by a dictaphone.

We interviewed 357 women or 54.09 % and 303 men or 45.91%.

For the standard of living with a low income was the most mentioned in four sectors, namely: Plateau or 68.18%; Sokoura or 51.82%; Dougoukoro or 50.91%; Hèrèmakono or 48.18% and the average income was the most mentioned in two sectors namely: Golf or 44.55% and ACI or 40.00%.

Fever (hot body) with 59.70% was the most common sign followed by headache with 59.39% and vomiting with 46.52%. The mosquito bite was the most mentioned either 67.12% of participants, followed by mosquito bites and food consumption with 12.73%. Most of the participants had a mosquito net that is 76.82%.

The first place of seeking care was self-medication with respectively 42.12% followed by consultation in a health centre with respectively 33.33%.

The mosquito net was the most used means with 45.76%.

The population of Baco-Djicoroni perceived malaria as a serious deadly disease and attributed the disease mostly to mosquito bites and therefore mostly used mosquito nets impregnated with insecticides to prevent it.

Keywords: **Malariae, Knowledge, Attitudes, Practices, Health Area, Prevention**

Questionnaire :

Knowledge, attitudes and practices of people in the Baco-Djicoroni health area regarding malaria prevention

Section 1: Socio-demographic characteristics

Questions

1. Residence (sector) :
2. Gender :
3. Age :
4. Nationality :
5. Marital status :
6. Level of study :
7. Profession :
8. Religion :
9. Ethnic group :
10. Standard of living :

Section 2: Knowledge about malaria, its transmission and prevention

11. Do you know what malaria is? yes ...no ...

If yes, how do you access information on malaria?

---

12. Do you know the signs of malaria? If so, name some.
13. How malaria is transmitted

---

14. Did you know that mosquitoes are the vectors of malaria? yes ... no...

If so, what kind of mosquito transmits malaria?

---

15. How many types of mosquito do you know

---

16. Do you know when the malaria mosquito bites (day or night) yes...no.

If yes, specify when

17. Do you know where the malaria mosquito lives? yes.no.

If yes, please specify

18. What preventive measures can be taken against malaria?

Section 3: Attitudes towards malaria and its prevention

19. Can anyone contract malaria?

I totally disagree. Disagree... I agree. Strongly agree.

Justify your answer

---

20. Are only children and pregnant women at risk?

Strongly disagree. I disagree. I agree. Totally agree.

Explain your answer

---

21. What would you do if you were faced with a case of malaria?
22. a) Use of the health centre

1- Yes / /2- No / /

22.b) Use of traditional healers

1- Yes / /2- No / /

22.c) Self-medication

1- Yes / /2- No / /

22. Malaria is a life-threatening disease?

Strongly disagree... I disagree... Agree... Totally agree...

Justify your answer

---

23. Can sleeping under a mosquito net at night prevent malaria?
Totally disagree. I disagree. Agree. Totally agree.
Explain your answer

24. Could not using mosquito nets when there are fewer mosquitoes increase the risk of contracting malaria?
Totally disagree. I disagree. Agree. Totally agree.
Justify your answer

Section 4: Practices for preventing malaria

25. Do you have a mosquito net? yes .no.
If so, how many do you have?

26. How often do you sleep under a mosquito net?
Always OftenNever
Justify your answer

27. How often do members of your family sleep under a mosquito net?
Always OftenNever
Explain your answer

28. How often do you check your mosquito net for repair holes?
Always OftenNever
Justify your answer

29. How often do you use repellents?
Always OftenNever
Explain your answer

30. How often do you use sprinklers in your home?
Always OftenNever
Justify your answer

31. How often do you weed your yard and surrounding area?
Always OftenNever
Explain your answer

32. How often do you remove stagnant water from your yard and surrounding area?
AlwaysOftenNever
Justify your answer

Focus group interview guide

Introduction :

Hello, I'm a medical student and my name is

I'm working on my doctoral thesis in medicine on malaria: knowledge, attitudes and practices of people in the Baco-Djicoroni health area regarding malaria prevention.

I'd like to find out about your knowledge, attitudes and practices when it comes to preventing malaria. There are no wrong answers, all answers are right and will help us to get to know and understand you better so that we can work better together.

Your comments and names will remain completely anonymous and strictly confidential.

You are free to participate and to withdraw from the interview at any time. I remain at your entire disposal for any further information or clarification you may require on points you have not understood.

Focus group recording sheet

N°	THEMES	SUB-THEMES

1	Knowledge of malaria	Can you tell me how you recognise that someone has a problem? malaria? Does malaria present differently in children and adults? Is there more than one term for malaria? What causes malaria? Do all mosquitoes transmit malaria? malaria? What should I do to protect myself against malaria?
2	Attitudes in the event of malaria	What would you do if you were faced with a case of malaria? Who would you make sleep under the mosquito net if there was only one in the house?
3	Practices in the event of malaria	Can you tell us what to do when faced with a case of malaria? Do you think it's necessary to sleep under an insecticide-treated mosquito net?

Thank you for your participation !!!!!!!

Certificates in research ethics

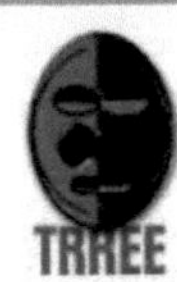

Zertifikat Certificado
Certificat Certificate

Promouvoir les plus hauts standards éthiques dans la protection des participants à la recherche biomédicale
Promoting the highest ethical standards in the protection of biomedical research participants

Certificat de formation - Training Certificate

Ce document atteste que - this document certifies that

Ramata yakare Traore

a complété avec succès - has successfully completed

Introduction to Research Ethics

du programme de formation TRREE en évaluation éthique de la recherche
of the TRREE training programme in research ethics evaluation

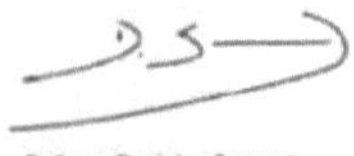

Release Date: 2020/03/12

Professeur Dominique Sprumont
Coordinateur TRREE Coordinator

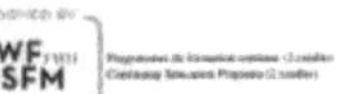

Foederatio Pharmaceutica Helvetiae FPH Programmes de formation postgraduée et continue

Ce programme est soutenu par · This program is supported by

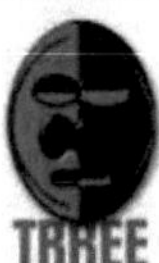

Zertifikat Certificado
Certificat Certificate

Promouvoir les plus hauts standards éthiques dans la protection des participants à la recherche biomédicale
Promoting the highest ethical standards in the protection of biomedical research participants

Certificat de formation - Training Certificate

Ce document atteste que - this document certifies that

Ramata yakare Traore

a complété avec succès - has successfully completed

Research Ethics Evaluation

du programme de formation TRREE en évaluation éthique de la recherche
of the TRREE training programme in research ethics evaluation

Release Date: 2020/03/12

Professeur Dominique Sprumont
Coordinateur TRREE Coordinator

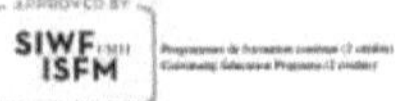

Foederatio Pharmaceutica Helvetiae FPH Programmes de formation postgraduée et continue

Ce programme est soutenu par · This program is supported by

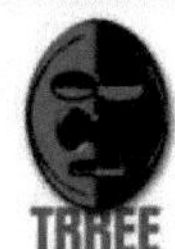

Zertifikat Certificado
Certificat Certificate

Promouvoir les plus hauts standards éthiques dans la protection des participants à la recherche biomédicale
Promoting the highest ethical standards in the protection of biomedical research participants

Certificat de formation - Training Certificate

Ce document atteste que - this document certifies that

Ramata yakare Traore

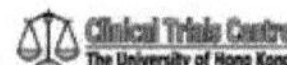

a complété avec succès - has successfully completed

Informed Consent

du programme de formation TRREE en évaluation éthique de la recherche
of the TRREE training programme in research ethics evaluation

Release Date: 2020/03/16

Professeur Dominique Sprumont
Coordinateur TRREE Coordinator

SIWF ISFM

Foederatio Pharmaceutica Helvetiae FPH Programmes de formation postgraduée et continue

Ce programme est soutenu par - This program is supported by

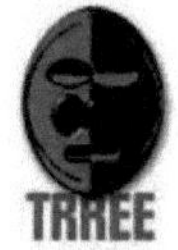

Zertifikat Certificado
Certificat Certificate

Promouvoir les plus hauts standards éthiques dans la protection des participants à la recherche biomédicale
Promoting the highest ethical standards in the protection of biomedical research participants

Certificat de formation - Training Certificate

Ce document atteste que - this document certifies that

Ramata yakare Traore

Clinical Trials Centre
The University of Hong Kong

a complété avec succès - has successfully completed

Good Clinical Practice (GCP-E6(R2) 2016)

du programme de formation TRREE en évaluation éthique de la recherche
of the TRREE training programme in research ethics evaluation

Release Date: 2020/03/16

Professeur Dominique Sprumont
Coordinateur TRREE Coordinator

SIWF ISFM

Foederatio Pharmaceutica Helvetiae FPH Programmes de formation postgraduée et continue

Ce programme est soutenu par - This program is supported by

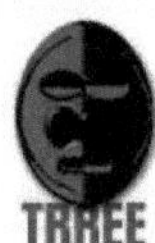

Zertifikat

Certificado

Certificat

Certificate

Promouvoir les plus hauts standards éthiques dans la protection des participants à la recherche biomédicale
Promoting the highest ethical standards in the protection of biomedical research participants

Certificat de formation - Training Certificate

Ce document atteste que - this document certifies that

Clinical Trials Centre
The University of Hong Kong

Ramata yakare Traore

a complété avec succès - has successfully completed

HIV Vaccine Trials

du programme de formation TRREE en évaluation éthique de la recherche
of the TRREE training programme in research ethics evaluation

Release Date: 2020/03/16

Professeur Dominique Sprumont
Coordinateur TRREE Coordinator

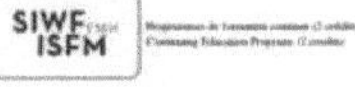

Foederatio Pharmaceutica Helvetiae

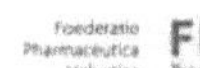

Programmes de formation postgraduée et continue

Ce programme est soutenu par - This program is supported by :

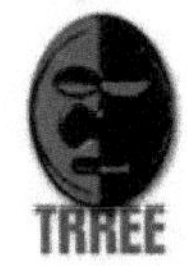

Zertifikat

Certificado

Certificat

Certificate

Promouvoir les plus hauts standards éthiques dans la protection des participants à la recherche biomédicale
Promoting the highest ethical standards in the protection of biomedical research participants

Certificat de formation - Training Certificate

Ce document atteste que - this document certifies that

Clinical Trials Centre
The University of Hong Kong

Ramata yakare Traore

a complété avec succès - has successfully completed

Adolescent Involvement in HIV Prevention Trials

du programme de formation TRREE en évaluation éthique de la recherche
of the TRREE training programme in research ethics evaluation

Release Date: 2020/03/16

Professeur Dominique Sprumont
Coordinateur TRREE Coordinator

SIWF ISFM

Foederatio Pharmaceutica Helvetiae

FPH

Programmes de formation postgraduée et continue

Ce programme est soutenu par - This program is supported by :

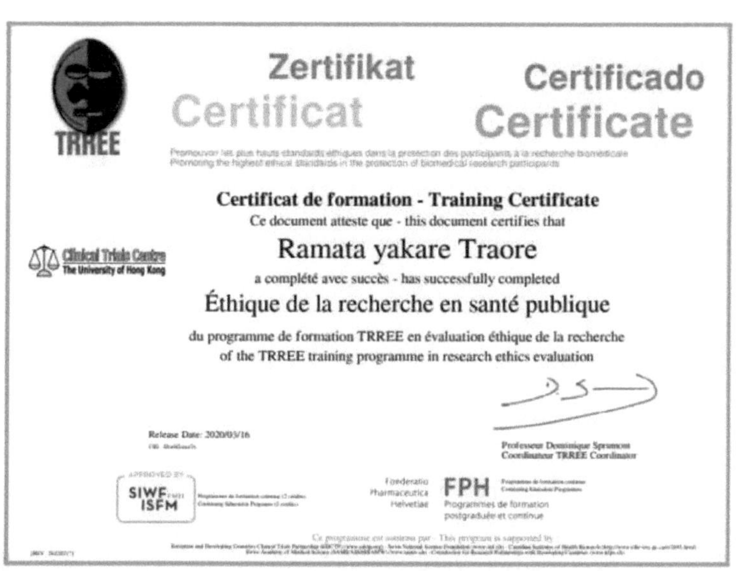

Zertifikat

Certificado

Certificat

Certificate

TRREE

Certificat de formation - Training Certificate

Ce document atteste que - this document certifies that

Ramata yakare Traore

a complété avec succès - has successfully completed

Éthique de la recherche en santé publique

du programme de formation TRREE en évaluation éthique de la recherche

of the TRREE training programme in research ethics evaluation

Clinical Trials Centre
The University of Hong Kong

Release Date: 2020/03/16

Professeur Dominique Sprumont
Coordinateur TRREE Coordinator

SIWF ISFM

Foederatio Pharmaceutica Helvetiae

FPH

Programmes de formation postgraduée et continue

Language transcription certificate (Bamanankan)

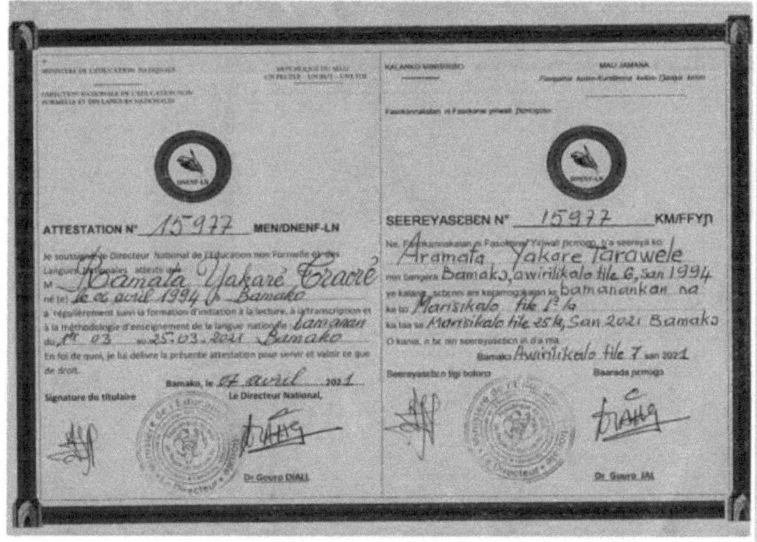

ATTESTATION N° 15977 MEN/DNENF-LN

Je soussigné, le Directeur National de l'Education non Formelle et des Langues Nationales atteste que

M Ramata Yakaré Traoré

né(e) le 06 avril 1994 à Bamako

a régulièrement suivi la formation d'initiation à la lecture, à la transcription et à la méthodologie d'enseignement de la langue nationale bamanan

du 1er 03 au 25.03.2021 Bamako

En foi de quoi, je lui délivre la présente attestation pour servir et valoir ce que de droit.

Bamako, le 07 avril 2021

Signature du titulaire

Le Directeur National,

Dr Gouro DIALL

SEEREYASƐBƐN N° 15977 KM/FFYɲ

Aramata Yakare Tarawele

min bangera Bamakɔ, awirilikalo tile 6, san 1994

bamanankan na

Marisikalo tile 1ɲ la

Marisikalo tile 25 la, San 2021 Bamakɔ

Bamakɔ Awirilikalo tile 7 san 2021

Baarada ɲɛmɔgɔ

Dr Gouro JAL

HIPPOCRATIC OATH

In the presence of the Masters of this Faculty, of my dear fellow students, before
the effigy of Hippocrates, I promise and swear, in the name of the supreme
being, to be
faithful to the laws of honour and probity in the practice of medicine.
I will give my care free of charge to the needy and will never demand a salary
above my work. I will not participate in any clandestine sharing of fees.
My eyes shall not see what goes on in the house, my
tongue shall not speak of the secrets entrusted to
me, and my status shall not serve to corrupt morals or encourage crime.
corrupt morals or encourage crime.
I will not allow considerations of religion, nation or race to
come between my duty and my patient.
I will maintain absolute respect for human life from the moment of conception.
Even under threat, I will not allow my medical knowledge to be used against the
laws of humanity.
against the laws of humanity.
Respectful and grateful to my Masters, I will give back to their children
the instruction I received from their fathers.
May men esteem me if I am faithful to my promises, and may
I be shamed and despised by my colleagues if I fail to keep them.

I swear!!!

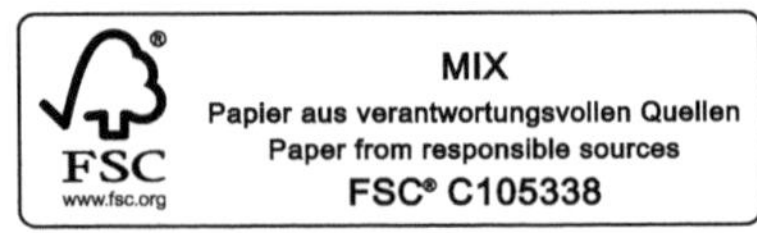

Printed by Books on Demand GmbH, Norderstedt / Germany